Woman
BOOK OF
SUCCESSFUL
SLIMMING

PAUL HAMLYN

LONDON · NEW YORK · SYDNEY · TORONTO

© Copyright Odhams Books 1966
Revised and reprinted 1970

Published by

THE HAMLYN PUBLISHING GROUP LIMITED

LONDON · NEW YORK · SYDNEY · TORONTO

Hamlyn House, Feltham, Middlesex, England

SBN 600 72994 x

PRINTED IN HONG KONG
BY THE CONTINENTAL PRINTING CO. LTD.

CONTENTS

Introduction: Why we wrote this book

The editors wish to point out that all information regarding slimming products was checked—for accuracy and availability—at the time of going to press. Later market changes may mean the introduction of new aids or the withdrawal of others.

WHY WE WROTE THIS BOOK

WE LIVE IN A FATTY LAND, a nation in which over half the adult population is estimated to be overweight. And if we continue to follow the pattern of other affluent countries, all the indications are that we shall continue to get fatter.

Does this matter?

WOMAN magazine, along with almost every medical expert in the land, believe that it does. And this book is dedicated to war on fat.

We have been waging this campaign against excess weight for many years now in the pages of our magazine. And as the largest and most influential women's journal in this country, we have felt it our duty to take the lead.

Our WOMAN diets have become famous. Our basic policy has never changed. We believe in making dieting as interesting, exciting and easy as possible. If we can make a diet fun to follow—then we have really scored a success. Because the important thing is this: if you are overweight, you should follow a diet that is stimulating and easy enough to lead you to complete slimming success. A diet that will work for *you*, as an individual.

But behind the attractive trimmings, we always insist that our diets are based on the soundest, most up-to-date medical principles; our own experts are working hand-in-hand with the leading nutritional and medical specialists in the country.

Slimming has ceased to be a joke. In recent years excess weight has been recognized as a great threat to health—and, in fact, a killer. We have asked a doctor to explain this to you in more detail at the end of this introduction.

But if you don't believe him, or us, try checking with the life insurance companies. See how your premiums go up if you are overweight.

To discover to what extent overweight affects life expectancy, a group of insurance companies carried out some special research. This showed that there is an increase of eight per cent in the average death rate of people 10 lbs. overweight, and twenty-eight per cent in those with an excess 30 lbs. When the excess weight reaches 50 lbs. this figure rises to fifty-six per cent.

Your health must always be the first factor for consideration. But being women ourselves, with an expert knowledge of other women through our contact with millions of readers, we are concerned with other aspects of slimming too.

We honestly believe that the loss of a stone or two can change a life in many exciting ways. We have seen this happen, because as part of our research we regularly take a group of readers under our wing for personal diet supervision.

This part of our work gives us real pleasure. Who doesn't like to play fairy godmother? Starting from the chrysalis of a heavy, and often unattractive, fairly lifeless woman, we delight in seeing a smart, self-assured, and highly attractive person emerge.

Excess weight, we are convinced, hampers the mind as well as the body. Fat so often leads to a built-in inferiority complex in women—a "well, what's the use" attitude to life in general.

Oddly enough, people often tend subconsciously to associate fatness in women with dullness, and a sleek figure with an alert mind. And perhaps there is some basis of truth in this feeling.

The woman who escapes from a hampering mountain of flesh often emerges to spread her wings in all directions.

There are so many advantages in being slim. Modern fashion is designed for the sleek shape; any overweight person out shopping will tell you that there is nothing "jolly" about being fat.

Modern high-pace living is geared to streamlined shapes in people as well as planes and cars. It is hard to keep up if you are carrying the handicap of one or two extra stone.

So far, in the pages of our magazine, we have had to ask you to take our slimming methods very much on trust. We have had to say: "Look, take our word for it, this is the best method," because there is not always the space to delve into detailed reasons.

We know that our readers have been largely content to rely on our reputation for integrity. And, of course, by following our diets they have been able to prove their effectiveness for themselves.

But at last, this book gives us the opportunity to tell you the full facts. Between these pages you will be able to learn exactly why we firmly believe that our own slimming methods are the best.

You will learn everything you need to know about slimming, from the reasons for your now being overweight, to the choice of clothes and foundations for the new slim figure which can very soon be yours. And having told you how to get slim, we don't neglect to tell you how you can *stay* slim, once and for all.

There are many reasons why this book is timely, and answers an urgent need for knowledge on this vital subject. Today, there's an increased awareness of the dangers of excess weight. And around a general desire to tackle this problem, there has grown a large industry.

Manufacturers by the dozen have turned their factories over to the production of slimming aids. Some are helpful and reputable. Others, we are sorry to say, are based on little more than wishful thinking.

The modern overweight woman has become easy prey to the "miracle men" with their useless inventions. Usually they are harmless. But a slimming aid that fails often destroys a woman's confidence. It convinces her, quite mistakenly, that she never can be slim.

As weight worries grow, we fully expect the slimming industry to grow with them. But by arming you with the true facts now, we can equip you to sort your way through the fiction.

In this book we give you all the help that we possibly can to lead you to the many rewards of being slim. We believe that we can convince and encourage you, and lead you to the easiest and most effective methods of slimming.

TURN THE PAGE FOR A DOCTOR'S POINT OF VIEW

A DOCTOR WRITES:

Perhaps the best way I can bring home to you the dangers of excess weight is by this one startling fact: Many more people die of overweight than of that great modern scourge—lung cancer.

This may shock you, and will almost certainly surprise you. And it is true that few death certificates would list "excess weight" as the actual cause of death.

But so often that extra fat, with all the increased strain that it imposes on the heart, arteries and other parts of the body, is the true culprit behind an illness. The health problems it can help to cause range from the relatively trivial—perhaps just shortage of breath and lack of energy—to the fatal.

Here are just some of the more serious illnesses which are more common in overweight people than slim people: arthritis, diabetes, brain haemorrhage, high blood pressure, inflammation of the gall bladder, cirrhosis of the liver, hernias, arteriosclerosis, kidney disease.

Overweight people are much more subject to life's little discomforts, like tiredness and aching feet, heat rashes, pains in the joints and insomnia. Statistics have shown that they are also more likely to have accidents, and they often face greater danger in the operating theatre than people of normal weight.

I won't go on—although I could for a considerable time. My object is not to depress you. But the facts must be faced.

By carrying around excessive weight you are making your bodily organs do excessive work. And the strain is likely to tell sooner or later.

Happily, I can end on a cheerful note by telling you of the wonderful health improvements that doctors so often see in people who were once fat, and have now managed to become slim. A new feeling of fitness and well-being becomes obvious. High blood pressure usually comes down. Those who have diabetes often find that their condition improves, sometimes even to a point where they can given up insulin.

As a doctor, I am concerned more with your health than with your appearance. And I do believe that sensible slimming is more than worth while on health grounds alone. If you are overweight now, I hope that you will take firm steps to correct this health danger in the very near future.

PART I

"You shall be yet fairer than you are."

WILLIAM SHAKESPEARE *(Antony and Cleopatra)*

"There is no doubt that people are interested in over-weight and most of them know its long-term dangers . . ."

THE PRACTITIONER *(March, 1963)*

CHAPTER 1
ARE YOU OVER-WEIGHT?

THIS BOOK is especially intended for the 60 per cent of British women who are—so a slimming-food manufacturer's survey tells us!—overweight. We hope it will also be of interest to slim women who may be concerned with the weight problems of some member of the family, and look-ahead people who want to make sure they stay slim.

But the first thing to decide is whether you belong to the overweight 6 out of every 10 (or, if you're a man, the overweight 7 out of every 10).

Yet surely, you might think, if a person should be overweight she can't fail to know it?

Oddly enough, inquiries suggest this is often not the case. According to a survey carried out by an opinion poll, only 32 per cent of the adult population, less than half of those who were overweight, realized that they weighed too much.

Having quoted these figures, we must add that we take them only as a loose indication of the problem. Because of basic differences in bones and muscles of body structure it is, for instance, impossible to say that the weight of absolutely every woman who is 5 ft. 4 in. tall should be 9 stone 2 lbs.

In marginal cases, one would have to consider many aspects of the individual to decide whether she was, in fact, carrying too much fat. And it would be difficult for any survey to take all of these aspects into account.

But the figures are impressive enough to make it clear that many people don't realize they are fatter than they should be. Why is this?

THAT "NORMAL" FIGURE

Well, obviously the reason is that many of us have different ideas on what is "normal" weight. These are coloured very much by the life we lead.

If you happen to be a middle-aged housewife of

reasonable proportions and your friends are mainly overweight middle-aged housewives, you may well feel that you are fairly slim.

But if you were to take an office job and work with young girls with sleek figures you might conceivably change your mind. By comparison you might now seem to be quite plump.

If you were to come and work at WOMAN, and see the constant procession of model girls, who have kitten hips and no more than 32 in. busts, that passes through our offices, you would probably decide that you were grossly overweight, even if you were almost skinny.

So you see, we tend to measure ourselves against the people we see around us. And this is not always the best and surest guide. So let's see now if we can find a better one.

THE GIRL YOU WERE

One of the first things to consider is: Are you fatter than you used to be?

Many people take it for granted that they will automatically gain weight as they grow older. And for a variety of reasons, in particular a decrease in physical activity, many people do so. But it does not follow that this is the right or even the natural thing for them.

Middle-aged spread is not inevitable. It can be avoided and it can be beaten. We have helped thousands of middle-aged women to slim on WOMAN Special-Design Diets. Excess weight in middle and older years is just as injurious to health as it is in youth—more so, in some ways.

So, if you are now over forty, look back to the girl that you used to be. If once upon a time you weighed 9 stone and you now weigh 11 stone, you can take it that you are now getting on for nearly 2 stone overweight. You can allow yourself 4 or

5 lbs. generosity in deference to your years if you wish. But this still means that you have many pounds to lose to achieve your own ideal proportions for health and looks.

Of course, this kind of calculation does not work for the young, nor for every older person. Some people have always been overweight. As you will learn later in this book, however, this rarely means that they need continue to be overweight. But at this stage they have probably become very accustomed to their extra fat and may not be really aware of it.

LOOK AND TOUCH TESTS

Unless you are already well aware that you are overweight, give your body a thoroughly frank appraisal. Lie down flat on your back, Is your tummy flat, or even slightly concave? It should be. Keep in this position and see if you can place a ruler at your side: to touch both your ribs and hip-bone—i.e. no spare tire.

Now stand up and measure round your chest (just beneath the breasts) and around your waist. There ought to be at least a few inches' difference in these measurements. If there's only one or two, it is another indication that you are carrying around excess flesh.

Can you gather handfuls of flesh by pinching yourself? Try this, particularly on the area between your bust and your waist.

Quite honestly, it isn't difficult to see if you're overweight, once you've accepted that you might be—even if you're a tiddler compared to Mrs. Jones next door. And once you've realized that age is no alibi for extra inches.

However, most people actually like to be able to climb onto the scales and compare their weight against an "ideal" weight, so we have compiled a height-and-weight chart for you, which you see below. But it is important to realize that this works only as a *rough guide* to help you to estimate the size of your own weight problem.

READING YOUR WEIGHT CHART Against each height we have given weights for small, average and large bone structure. The size of bones does make a difference to weight. But not as much as some people like to imagine. Even the largest, heaviest bones could not account for more than 10 lbs. excess weight.

You can tell whether you are small-boned or large-boned by considering your hands and feet,

IDEAL WEIGHT CHART
(Women)
(Add approx. 3–4 lbs. for indoor clothes)

Height Without Shoes	Weight Small Frame		Weight Medium Frame		Weight Large Frame	
ft. in.	st.	lbs.	st.	lbs.	st.	lbs.
4 9	7	4	7	9	8	4
4 10	7	7	7	12	8	7
4 11	7	10	8	1	8	10
5 0	7	13	8	4	8	13
5 1	8	2	8	7	9	2
5 2	8	5	8	10	9	5
5 3	8	7	8	13	9	8
5 4	8	10	9	2	9	12
5 5	8	13	9	5	10	2
5 6	9	3	9	9	10	6
5 7	9	6	9	13	10	9
5 8	9	9	10	3	10	13
5 9	9	13	10	7	11	3
5 10	10	3	10	12	11	7
5 11	10	6	11	2	11	11

shoulders and wrists. If, for instance, you take a very small size in gloves and shoes, if your wrists are slim and shoulders small, you are small-boned, and should weigh a few pounds less than the average person of your height.

If, on the other hand, you take large sizes in shoes and gloves and you have fairly broad shoulders and wide wrists, you are large-boned. You must expect to weigh a few pounds more than the average person of your height.

Your bone size may be anywhere between the two extremes catered for by our table. So if you feel you are just "fairly" small-boned, or just "fairly" large-boned it's up to you to adjust it by a pound or two.

Another factor it might be necessary for you to take into consideration is muscles.

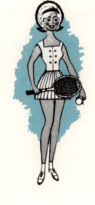

If you are still at school or college and you take physical exercise regularly, or if sport happens to be one of your hobbies, your muscles will be more developed than those of the average person. They might well account for a few pounds extra weight. So take this into account when you compare yourself against our tables.

But if you cheat, and provide yourself with any unjustified alibis for your weight, remember that you are cheating only yourself. You may convince yourself that all that weight is due to huge bones and whopping muscles, but you're very unlikely to convince anyone else. Even that would not matter so much if it were not for the fact that excess fat is downright unhealthy.

IF IN DOUBT

In giving advice to the "Shall I, Shan't I?" person who is considering a diet we usually reverse the advice that we would give to the hesitant girl considering whether or not to marry. For to the reluctant bride we would say: "If in doubt—don't" while to you, the hesitant slimmer, we can safely say: "If in doubt—*DO*!"

Because on a WOMAN diet you have nothing to lose but your excess poundage!

In particular, the average-speed diets that we give in this book just constitute a pattern of eating that any normal, healthy person, whether slim or fat, could safely follow.

However, we don't honestly believe that very many of you will still be labouring under any great doubt about your excess weight.

So let's get straight down to business.

Start by asking yourself these questions:
   1. **Am I overweight because I tend to be rather greedy?**
   2. **Am I overweight for the simple reason that my parents were fat?**
   3. **Do I blame my weight problem on my glands?**
   4. **Am I overweight because my body retains too much water?**
   5. **Did I gain my extra weight during pregnancy?**
   6. **Am I just suffering from "puppy fat"?**

CHAPTER 2
WHY YOU PUT ON WEIGHT

NOW YOU MAY KNOW you are overweight. And having answered the questions at the end of the previous chapter, you probably feel that you know just why you are.

But here we must confess to having led you on a little. It is highly unlikely that your weight problems are indeed caused by greed, heredity, glands or liquid retention, or even largely by pregnancy or puppy fat. These are popular and understandable alibis, with which people tend to "comfort" themselves. But, as we shall see, they are very often misleading.

You'll agree that to find a cure for almost any problem it is first necessary to discover the true cause. And in dealing with the problems of excess weight this means wading through a whole lot of widely accepted but mistaken notions to get at the real truth.

Let's see how well most of those generally accepted "causes of overweight" really stand up to a thorough examination.

GREED— THE SECRET GUILT

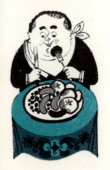

Is the woman who carries around two or three extra stone simply guilty of gluttony?

The dictionary defines a glutton as "one who eats to excess" and in a strictly medical sense, as we shall see later, that tag could be linked to the overweight woman.

But what about the everyday sense of the word? Here we usually visualize the glutton as a greedy soul obsessed with eating, knowing no decent bounds to appetite.

Surely that can't be you! We are quite sure that it isn't. And it certainly isn't a description of the hundreds of overweight women who have come to WOMAN for help.

On the contrary, in our own experience the

typical overweight woman cares little about her own meals. So often she is a busy housewife absorbed in feeding and caring for her family, just grabbing "anything that is going" to feed herself; almost certainly she misses a proper breakfast and snatches a cup of tea and "a bite of something" for elevenses.

When she knows for a fact that she rarely eats more than a couple of slices of toast for breakfast, and seldom has time for more than a sandwich at lunchtime, she finds those pounds just plain puzzling. So she looks for, and often finds, one of those special "causes of overweight" which we are about to discuss.

The secret fears that they might be guilty of greed lie at the back of the minds of many women. That is why one of the first things they rush to tell us is:

"I'm not a great eater, you know—I hardly eat any very big meals. I'm sure I don't eat more than most people!"

We believe them. We believe you. In sheer bulk the overweight woman is often not eating more than many other people who manage to remain slim. We promise faithfully that the words "greed" and "gluttony" will not be mentioned again in this book.

DON'T BLAME MOTHER

Perhaps that heredity factor is against you. Your mother is fat, your father is fat, even your grandmother was fat. What possible chance have you of being slim?

It seems to be just your bad luck that you come from a fatty family. A survey has shown that when both parents are overweight, seventy five per cent of the children are overweight (and when neither of the parents is overweight, only nine per cent of

10

the children become overweight). And statistics, they say, are things you can't argue about. Or are they...? Before you throw in the towel, burn this book, and let out another set of seams, take a look at the story of Susan:

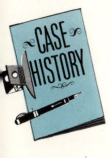

Susan was a personal friend of a WOMAN staff member, so we knew a good deal about her before she came to consult us about her figure problems. In fact, we are pretty certain that she wouldn't have come at all if she hadn't been invited. Because Susan considered herself to be a fairly hopeless case.

If you had a glimpse at the snapshots in the family photograph album, you would very soon see why she was despondent about her $12\frac{1}{2}$ stone figure. Susan's sister was huge. We don't know her exact weight but guesses would start well over 15 stone. Her mother was almost as fat, and her father was, to say the least, "portly".

Susan considered that she had just inherited this weight problem and was stuck with it. And quite frankly, she didn't make any great effort to do much about it.

We have said that the overweight woman is often not eating more than other people who manage to remain slim. But this wasn't so in Susan's case. This girl really loved her food, man-sized helpings of potatoes and spaghetti, pies and puds, the lot. Well, what was the use? thought Susan. She was going to be fat anyway, so might as well enjoy herself . . .

If we hadn't had her husband on our side (contrary to the widely prevalent idea, we find that husbands are usually extremely keen to help their wives to slim) we would probably never have been able to get Susan to start on a diet. But diet she did—and there was just no stopping her after the first week of her new regime when, to her utter astonishment, she lost a stunning 7 lbs. in weight.

Susan in fact lost weight (2½ stone eventually) even more rapidly than girls from slimmer families. And she is not an isolated example, but a typical one.

In our long experience we have invariably found that women from overweight families can slim just as swiftly as any one else. Then what explains those statistics? Why is it that a general pattern of overweight definitely tends to run in families?

Well, in the first place, the medical experts do acknowledge the fact that it is possible to inherit a large frame—the basic bonework of the body. That can account for a little of the weight, but not of the actual fat. It is also possible to inherit a tendency to your own particular proportions—largish thighs, a more ample bust than hips, or vice versa.

But medical evidence, plus our own repeated proof of how easily that so called "inherited bulk" can be shed, has shown quite clearly that no-one is condemned to be fat simply because of the weight of her parents.

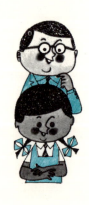

What children of overweight parents so often inherit—and this is the whole key to those statistics—is a tendency to bad eating habits. From the time they are tiny tots they have been trained to eat in the way which has almost certainly been responsible for their parents' weight problems.

We're coming nearer the truth of the matter now. Bad eating habits are something we are going to learn a lot about. But for the meantime rest assured that even if you come from the longest line of fatties ever to weigh down a family tree, you can still be slim.

The glandular factor is often discussed as a possible cause of excess weight. It is quite true that if the thyroid gland is not working correctly the body can have a tendency to produce excess fat; and other glands like the pituitary and the suprarenal can also be responsible for this.

But instances in which overweight is directly caused by gland problems are very rare indeed. We have come across only one or two in all our years of contact with overweight women, and all our slimmers are given a very thorough health check by a medical specialist before they ever embark on a diet.

We can safely say that it is highly unlikely that you are overweight because of your glands. If you were, other symptoms easily recognizable by a doctor would show themselves. And even then there would be no need for despair, because often this condition can be treated under medical supervision.

If, by the time you have read this book and discovered the true culprits behind most extra inches, you can still say quite firmly: "But those just don't apply to me"—then do have a medical check-up. It is a wise step, anyway, if you are in any doubt about your health.

But the vast majority of us can just leave our glands to look after themselves—and look for more simple reasons for this extra weight.

Many people believe that they are gaining weight simply because they are retaining too much liquid in the body. That is why they try to

13

cut down on their drinking, and, if they follow the theory through a little further, their consumption of salt.

If we consider the facts we will see where this idea springs from. Three quarters of the body consists of water. It is essential to have just the right amount of water in the blood and between the body cells, and one of the things which regulates the amount is common salt.

If for some reason too much salt accumulates in your body, water accumulates with it and you become overweight and ill.

But notice that we said "ill". All healthy bodies even fat ones, perfectly regulate their correct amount of salt and water by excreting the excess of both. We all take in very much more than we need of both in normal eating and drinking.

So it's no use saying: "I'm fine—my body just retains rather too much water and that makes me put on weight!" You wouldn't be fine at all, if that were genuinely the case, and you would be in need of medical treatment.

Again, this condition is rare. So for nearly all overweights, here's another "good cause" that can be forgotten.

POUNDS THAT BABY BROUGHT

Ah, here's one that we can't dismiss so easily You blame pregnancy for overweight. This time you are working on facts, not theories. You know jolly well that before your first pregnancy you weighed nine stone, and afterwards you were nearer ten. And the same sort of thing happened with the second baby.

Yes, its quite true that during pregnancy the body does tend to store fat, due to a change in glandular activity (one case where the glands can be given part of the blame). And most of us are also aware that these days most doctors are keen that we should keep this fat-gaining tendency in check. But few women manage to emerge from pregnancy without having gained at least a few extra pounds on the way. Those of us who've tried it know how hard it is.

It would be no exaggeration to say that at least seventy-five per cent of the over-thirties who consult WOMAN about slimming have gained the bulk of their extra poundage during child-bearing. Or at least, as one of them put it: "That was the beginning of the rot!"

But here is another thing that we have proved over and over again, and which all medical evidence would support: it is no more difficult to shed pounds that you have gained through pregnancy than it is to shed the pounds you have gained through any other cause.

So although it is quite understandable that you gained some of those excess pounds at the time— can you really blame pregnancy two, or ten, years later?

Take heart, pregnancy may make you a little plumper at the time. It shouldn't, and certainly needn't, make you fatter ever after.

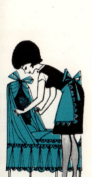

PUPPY FAT

We all know the teenager who groans about her podgy shape, and the comforting mother who tells her "Never mind dear, it's just your age. It's puppy fat, there's nothing you can do until you grow out of it!"

How right is the mother? Well, she is correct to the extent that her daughter's age is contributing to the problem. At the beginning of puberty new hormones begin to circulate in a young girl's body. These hormones are working at altering her contours and developing her adult shape. And in the

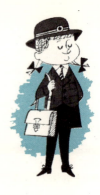

early stages they can, to put it simply, be a little haphazard and a little overgenerous in their distribution of fat.

Puppy fat is a serious problem to no-one but the teenager herself. Two or three years can seem an awfully long time, as all of us who used to be "the podgy girl" can remember.

Happily, something can be done about it by simply adjusting the regular eating habits. As you begin to learn more about WOMAN slimming methods you will realize why they are so safe and effective, even for teenagers.

THE REAL CAUSE OF EXCESS WEIGHT

Now that we know what *isn't* making us overweight, all that remains is to discover what, in fact is. And the answer is just this:

If you take in more food than you use you will put on weight.

This is easily understood by thinking of food in terms of the energy to which the body converts it.

The following three facts are the very heart of this whole slimming business.

If the amount of energy (food) that is being taken in is equal to the amount of energy (all effort and activity) that is being given out, the body will stay at the same weight.

If the amount of energy going in is in excess of that being used up, the body will convert the extra into fat for storage, and gain weight.

If the emount of energy going in is less than that being used up, the body will draw on stores of fat, and lose weight.

But how does that tie up with the statement made earlier in this chapter that the overweight woman is often not eating more than many other people who manage to remain slim?

Well, the other people may just be leading more

active lives, and are thus increasing their energy output. But even that need not be the final truth of the matter.

You see, your body is unique. Just as your face and features have much in common with, but much that is different from, other people's, so your body works in a basically similar yet slightly different way.

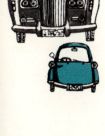

A Bentley and a Bubble Car, travelling at the same speed, over the same distance, would use up vastly different amounts of petrol. And similarly, two people doing exactly the same amount of work, even just breathing, might burn up vastly different amounts of food or energy.

The woman who is putting on weight is eating too much food for herself, but not necessarily too much food for her friend who has a higher metabolic (food-using) rate.

As Professor John Yudkin, one of the leading authorities on nutrition, puts it: "You will put on fat if you eat more than you use up. Overweight comes from over-eating. And over-eating need not mean a lot of food, but too much food, which still may be relatively little."

Now we are getting to the truth of the matter— but so far only half of the truth. Because there is another equally important factor that should be taken into account.

We know that the overweight woman is eating too much for her own body. But the next important question is: "Too much of what?"

Medical discoveries in very recent years have shown that while any type of food, if eaten to huge excess, could cause accumulation of fat, there are some foods which are, in practice, much greater fat producers than others.

You will learn all about this later when we

explain the research breakthrough that lies behind WOMAN dieting. But first it is important for you to understand why you overeat.

Ask yourself these questions:

1. **Have my eating habits** (choice of food, amount, routine) changed a great deal from those I learned as a youngster in my parents' home?

2. **Do I eat only** when I am hungry?

3. **Am I inclined** to eat more when I am worried or upset?

4. **Do I tend** to "punctuate" the day with little eating sessions—regarding "a cup of tea and . . ." as a nice natural break to work or boredom?

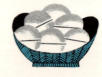

CHAPTER 3

WHAT MAKES US OVER-EAT?

IF A MODERN GOOD FAIRY decided to make a really practical wish over the cradle of a baby girl, she would grant her the gift of an always "perfectly adjusted appestat".

And with a single wave of her magic wand this good fairy would ensure that one lucky female, at least, never had to worry about puppy fat, middle-aged spread or spare tires, throughout the rest of her life.

The appestat is the part of the brain which controls the amount of food we feel like eating. It is the thought centre from which springs our desire for food.

If it is working perfectly, the appestat sees to it that we eat exactly the amount of food we need. It asks us to take in an extra quantity of food if we are doing more work than usual and less if for some reason we are not so active as we normally are.

But unfortunately, some appestats, like some characters, can be more easily coaxed away from the path of duty than others.

We have talked about the slim person who always eats a generous amount of food, yet doesn't put on weight because her body is the kind that uses up food rapidly.

But most of us also know the slim person who eats less than we do. She may actually want to eat more, and put on weight, but she can't seem to do it. When she has taken in enough for her own particular energy output, the thought of an extra portion does nothing but fill her with revulsion.

For that girl, the appestat is an unyielding dictator. But for the majority of us—those who can manage to put on that extra weight only too easily—the appestat has become over-indulgent

going to tend to throw our appestats slightly out of adjustment.

It is easy enough to tell someone to give up a pleasure—not always as easy to follow that advice. But we promise faithfully that it hurts only at first. Once the habit has been definitely broken, the appestat begins to work efficiently again. And when the appestat is boss there is no longer any great desire for "just for fun" eating.

EATING TO COMPENSATE

To some people, food is a symbol of love and security. They find it comforting. This is not surprising if you take another look back to childhood, and remember that the crying baby is often comforted by an extra or an earlier feed, the toddler who grazes his knee is often given a sweet as well as a kiss.

It is not at all unusual for a woman who has suffered an emotional shock—perhaps a broken marriage or bereavement—to put on a lot of weight in a short period of time. She turns to the chocolate box or biscuit tin for moments of comfort. In a way, she is also often trying subconsciously to fill a gap in her life by adding more food. The food is being used to compensate for something else.

Many people tend to over-eat during periods of worry, tension or unhappiness. Many more people over-eat just through sheer boredom— once again, they are subconsciously making an effort to "fill the gap".

The woman who is bored is not a happy or satisfied woman. She almost certainly lacks a feeling of fulfilment, and she is going to have to tackle these basic problems before trying to tackle the problem of her figure.

This point was brought home clearly to us by

Mrs. S., who looked as if she was to be one of our rare slimming failures. Not because she couldn't lose weight on a diet (we have never seen anyone fail for that reason) but because she just couldn't *keep* to a diet.

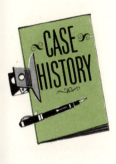

Mrs. S. was a woman in her late thirties, married to a successful business-man. They were a couple who had risen considerably in the world, and Mr. S. was all for them enjoying their new-found wealth.

They had a nice home, and a "daily" who came in regularly to do all the heavy work and keep it clean for them. But to their sorrow they had never had any children.

Mrs. S. did a certain amount of entertaining. But for the most part she found herself with time on her hands and, more often than not, felt a little bored with life.

She also found herself almost 2 stone overweight; that was why she came to see us.

Unlike most overweight women who have a real conviction that they are not over-eating, Mrs. S. herself had a fairly shrewd idea about the basic cause of her problem.

She admitted frankly to us that she did a great deal of eating in between meals. A break for coffee or tea and cakes helped to pass away the morning or the afternoon, and Mr. S. never forgot to bring her home the weekly box of chocolates.

With an equal frankness we told Mrs. S. that this would really have to stop. We could do nothing for her unless she could agree to cut out those sweet snacks.

She was very keen on losing weight. With her fortieth birthday looming so close ahead she had suddenly taken stock of herself. And she realized at this point that her weight was already giving her a matronly look, while some of her slimmer friends were still keeping their youthful appearance.

So Mrs. S. promised to be really firm with herself. We put her on a diet which had been geared as closely as was possible to her own will-power and personality. And off she went with great enthusiasm and determination to follow it strictly.

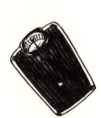

In the first week, Mrs. S. did quite well. She lost 4 lbs. and was, not surprisingly, very encouraged by this. Then in the second week she managed to lose another 2 lbs.

But the third week was a disappointment. She was barely 1 lb. down.

On the fourth week she didn't appear for her weight check: her husband telephoned to say that she had a bit of a cold.

After that she turned up spasmodically from time to time, to record only a very small loss, or none at all. And eventually Mrs. S. ceased her visits altogether.

That would have seemed to be the rather sad end to the story of Mrs. S. and her slimming. As she didn't even answer our letters all we could do was to close her file and write her off as a lost cause.

But, much to our surprise, more than a year later Mrs. S. suddenly came back into our lives with an unexpected phone call. She was awfully sorry about "just disappearing like that" she explained, obviously with considerable em-barrassment, but could she please have one more chance at dieting with us?

Frankly, we were a little dubious. We can take only a very small percentage of our readers under our wing for individual diet supervision, and it didn't seem quite fair to others to give one person a second chance.

However, we invited Mrs. S. around to have a chat with us about it.

As soon as she came into the room we could see that there was something different about her. She had a livelier look, and a much more enthusiastic approach.

"I'm a Mum now—well, a foster Mum at any rate!" she explained, and we learned how, under a local council scheme, she had taken two children in need of a temporary home.

Conversation got back inevitably to the failure of her previous diet.

"To be honest," said Mrs. S., "I just couldn't stop my between-meal eating. You see, I managed it for the first couple of weeks, but then I couldn't resist my snacks.

"I really felt that I was letting you down, after you had gone to so much trouble to help me, and I just didn't have the courage to admit it to you, face to face."

This was all very understandable. But what was it that made Mrs. S. feel she could react any differently now, we asked.

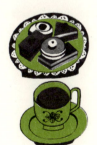

"Well, apart from anything else, I'm so busy that I hardly have time to sit down for tea and cakes," she told us. "I've lost a bit of weight already."

We felt there was another reason too: Mrs. S. had filled a gap in her life, and she was now a busy and happy person. She no longer needed to eat as a compensation.

This was a new Mrs. S. who, inadvertently, had got right to the root of her overweight problem, so we agreed she should slim with us again, and this time we were able to chalk up a complete success.

By telling the story of Mrs. S. we are not in the least suggesting that all childless women need to take on a family before they are able to slim successfully. All we are pointing out is that unhappiness and boredom can lead to bad eating habits, and that at times some new activities and interests can play an essential part in readjusting the appestat.

IN SEARCH OF A SOLUTION

Having read these three chapters you should now know if you are overweight, and why you are overweight. And the solution to your problem will have begun to make itself fairly clear. However, the claims of commercial interests and well-meaning friends may still suggest to you that there are a variety of solutions to this overweight problem.

So let's not ignore all these popular theories going the rounds.

Ask yourself these questions before reading the next chapter:
1. **Do I know of any other successful slimming methods besides dieting?**
2. **Have I tried them?**
3. **Did I lose weight?**

CHAPTER 4
THE "MIRACLE METHODS"

THE OVERWEIGHT WOMAN who comes to us for help often comes in search of a little magic.

We see the pattern repeated hundreds of times. The eager expectancy. The long discussion about pounds that gradually accumulated over the years. Then the let-down when we explain we're going to put her on a diet; just a sensible, balanced diet using everyday foods—no yak's milk or plovers' eggs, no pills, nothing sensational.

She rarely hides her disappointment.

"Oh, but diets just don't work for me," she tells us. "I've been trying them for years. And anyway, I eat very little as it is."

You will see now why in Chapter 2 we explored those "special reasons" for being overweight so thoroughly. If a woman mistakenly believes that there is some particular reason behind her extra inches—nothing so simple as just eating too much for her needs, or at least too much of the wrong foods—it is understandable that she is going to look for some very special solution. Unless she understands that her eating habits are the cause, she is hardly going to believe that changing them can be the only cure.

What's more, in search of her "special cure" she will become easy prey for anyone who can dream up some miracle fat-melting formula.

Even a highly intelligent woman is susceptible. She may be the type who can see at a glance through the extravagant claims of a doorstep salesman, or can cause difficulty for her M.P. with a really searching question. But present her with some "revolutionary" method of slimming, and the chances are she will swallow it.

Whole industries have been founded on slimming methods that just couldn't work.

The woman who falls for the "miracle methods"

isn't stupid. She's just human. Besieged on all sides by a mass of conflicting claims—drink this and the pounds will roll away, wear this and you'll be slimmer in a matter of days, try this marvellous new machine (there's never been anything like it) —she quite naturally plumps for the one which seems to demand the least effort or seems to present a solution to her own "special problem". And by this reckoning, the poor old diet, unless it claims to include some stupendous, never-before-discovered, lightning-slim ingredient, takes a decided last place.

Of course, all overweight women dabble with diets at some time or other. Many embark on them as often as heavy smokers give up cigarettes, and with about the same success! After a few days, or weeks, the diet is abandoned. Usually the diet itself is to blame, demanding too much effort for too little return. And now the would-be slimmer has another reason for feeling sure that diets just aren't any use for her. Well, she's tried it, hasn't she, and it didn't work . . .

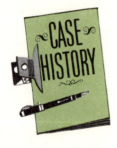

Mrs. P. who came to consult our WOMAN slimming experts was a fairly typical example—different only in that she expressed her views more frankly and forcibly than most. Aged forty-five, she was the wife of a Civil Servant, the mother of two children, and still continued her school-teaching career. A pretty firm, no-nonsense sort of woman, Mrs. P. We could tell that she didn't at all like having to ask advice on a subject like slimming. But she was a good 2 stone overweight and the breathlessness and tiredness this caused was proving a serious handicap in her busy life.

Mrs. P.'s attitude was almost aggressive when she first walked into our consulting room and the undercurrents were apparent. We were obviously being "challenged" to find a cure for her and, my goodness, it had better be convincing!

All seemed to be going well as Mrs. P. "thawed" a little under a sympathetic hearing. Here at least was someone who seemed to take her problem seriously, and be anxious to help. But when we suggested a diet the explosion came.

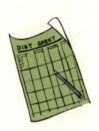

Mrs. P. stood up.

"If all you can offer is a diet I might as well go now and save your time and mine.

"My dear woman, if you knew the number of times I have tried to diet. And it just didn't do any good at all. If I could lose weight simply by dieting I wouldn't be bothering you."

It took a good ten minutes to sooth Mrs. P. down and persuade her to at least hear all of our point of view. Finally, we suggested:

"Well, why not try it our way for just a couple of weeks? If you don't lose weight you can come and show us just how wrong we are, and then we'll take it from there. But if you do lose weight, you win in any case."

Mrs. P. was a sporting woman, and a fair one. She went off determined to prove us wrong, and almost anxious to. But she kept strictly to the diet we gave her, and which she had thought far too generous in food anyway.

On her first weight check after one week she had lost $3\frac{3}{4}$ lbs. and on the following week she took off another 2 lbs.

We became great friends with Mrs. P. and she was a popular visitor as she called in week after week to record the loss of yet another 2 or 3 lbs. and eventually the whole tiring 2 stone.

As friends we were able to learn the real story of those previous "diets". Mrs. P. had been what we term a "starvation dieter". Every now and then, feeling quite desperate about her weight, she tried to put herself on a really spartan regime of eating. That usually consisted of missing out breakfast and lunch altogether. But often she just didn't have the will-power to get through to her evening meal on this fast, and would have to eat some biscuits, and perhaps a little fruit during the course of the day.

Her evening meal was quite sensible—she knew that potatoes and sweet things were fattening and kept to very small portions. But by bedtime she often still felt hungry and had to have cheese and biscuits or a sandwich for supper.

Results: too little food to keep Mrs. P. happy and satisfied. Yet too much of the wrong food—which you will learn more about later in this book—to allow her to lose weight.

No wonder that Mrs. P. nearly hit us when we suggested dieting to her.

In this chapter we want to prove to you, as we did to Mrs. P. that diets—but only the right balanced diets, of course—are the easiest way, the fastest way, the safest way, the *ONLY* way of losing weight permanently.

DOES EXERCISE HELP?

When you recall that the reason people put on weight is that they take in more units of energy in food than their bodies use up in activity, it is quite logical to assume that increased activity is the answer. Surely if you burn up more energy in exercise and sports you'll lose weight!

You can add to this the fact that many doctors believe the widespread overweight tendency in industrial countries is partly due to a decrease in physical activity.

We will ride in a car, bus or train instead of

walking or running. We often work with our brain or hands only. We relax by watching TV.

Right, then. Let's tackle this slimming business from the energy output end. Let's start by an hour's tennis or badminton, or half an hour's knees-bend-arms-stretch.

At the end of it you are probably feeling pretty puffed but fairly virtuous. You climb on the scales and may even find that you seem to have lost a little weight. But wait—remember that you have been perspiring more rapidly than usual. As you will realize, temporary water loss must mean temporary weight loss. You are probably feeling thirsty this very minute . . .

A little later in the day you can try the scales again, and this time you will find the weight-loss caused by that hectic bout of energy is hardly big enough to register. You are aware of something else too—a keen appetite.

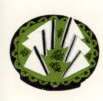

Perhaps you will cut yourself a sandwich right away, or you may help yourself to another potato at the next meal. That single sandwich, even a very slim one, or that potato, will undo—or more than undo—all the slimming progress that energetic exercise achieved.

Of course if you resisted the temptation to eat more for the rest of the day, or appeased your hunger with foods that were not readily convertible to body fat, the story would be different. But we've come the full circle here—we've come right back to what is in fact, *a diet*.

As a method of weight reduction, exercise alone is totally impractical. Even if you overlook that "increased appetite" factor it is a painfully slow method. The woman who wants to lose weight wants to lose it in months, not years.

But are the doctors talking complete nonsense

then, when they declare that lack of exercise is a contributing cause of excess weight?

Not at all. Exercise as a *preventative* measure must be considered in quite a different light from exercise as a quick cure.

The overweight middle-aged person often gains much of her extra weight slowly and gradually. An increase of just 2 lbs. a year from the time she's twenty-five means that when she's forty-five she's had a weight gain of *3 stone*.

Regular exercise could have tipped the balance, and prevented that annual 2 lb. gain—and so also that staggering 3 stone. There is evidence to suggest that when exercise is taken regularly over a long period, the appestat becomes adjusted to it, and there is none of that increase in hunger.

So we aren't against exercise. We're all for it because of its obvious benefits to health, and we have even included a chapter, with examples, on exercise in this book.

Exercise is particularly valuable to the slimmer because it firms her muscles while her diet melts the fat away. It makes sure that she will look young, lithe and slim. Not just slim.

But exercise alone can never be a successful slimming method.

"SWEATING IT OFF"

Points we have already discussed have probably given you a good idea, by now, that the popular "sweating it off" theory is just not going to "hold water". And yet—it *seems* so convincing.

You take a Turkish bath, you weigh yourself before you go in and, sure enough, when you weigh yourself again afterwards you *have* lost a pound or two.

But what the majority of people fail to do is weigh themselves again a few hours later. If they

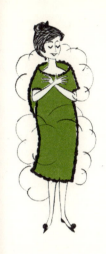

did, they'd almost certainly find that those lost pounds had mysteriously crept back again. It's quite simple, really: heavy perspiration reduces the liquid content of your body, and for a while you will weigh less. But, as you've learned, the body regulates its liquid content to a fairly set level. From your next drink or so it will retain liquid to put things back as they were. By being permanently thirsty you could weigh less—but could anything be much more unpleasant?

A jockey or boxer who must reduce to a certain weight for a race or fight will use this method for a few days. But he's aiming for a *temporary* weight loss, and knows his weight will go up again when he resumes normal life after the event.

The Turkish bath which has other real virtues, even if slimming is not one of them, is not the only "reducing method" based on the dehydration theory. Manufacturers have thought up other ways to make you perspire for the good of your figure.

Often women following these methods are advised to diet, too. That's a good idea. The dieting may slim you. Just perspiring won't.

CUTTING DOWN WATER AND SALT

If getting rid of more liquid from your body won't make you slim, it follows that taking in less liquid will have no permanent effect either.

Some people will tell you to drink less, to improve your figure. They are on the right track if they mean less alcohol, or less of any drink which has a fattening content. But if they mean less water (or other non-fattening drinks which you will be told about in connection with your WOMAN diet) they have got hold of quite the wrong idea.

Again, the only way to lose weight by this

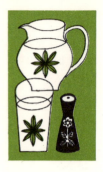

method would be to remain permanently thirsty.

The theory of salt reduction as a slimming method arises from the same misunderstanding. Salt helps your body to retain just the right amount of water, so the reduction of salt, they argue, must surely lead to the reduction of water-content and therefore of overall bulk.

But have you thought how difficult it would be to starve yourself of salt? The average person takes about ten times the amount of salt she needs in normal everyday eating. The excess does no harm to a healthy person, and is excreted by the body.

So to keep your body short of salt you would need to take less than a tenth of your normal amount. This wouldn't just mean cutting out the pinch at the side of your plate. It would mean cutting salt out of cooking, and abandoning all the high salt-content foods, like many types of fish.

Even if you were prepared for all this, salt starvation would not be wise on medical grounds.

You may have heard of an overweight friend who is cutting down salt on doctor's orders, but this is quite a different matter. Her excess weight is probably caused by a health problem, and cutting down on salt may be part of the treatment.

But for you, salt reduction is unlikely to provide any long-term solution to your weight problems.

We'll dispose of another small but persistent part of the dehydration theory here. People will tell you that toast is less fattening than bread.

Toast is bread minus some of its water content. So, for the purpose of slimming, whether you toast your bread or not matters not a jot.

LEMON JUICE

It is easy to see how the misconceptions which lead people to pin their slimming hopes on exercise or

VINEGAR AND SUCH-LIKE

dehydration arose. But here's another theory which is really based on nonsense.

Some people believe that if they take a certain thing—usually it's lemon juice or cider-vinegar—*in addition to* their normal food and drink, it will somehow magically melt their fat away.

No one has yet come up with any sound scientific suggestion as to why this should work. Because, of course, it doesn't work.

The reason is as simple as elementary mathematics. You can't subtract by addition. Nothing you eat or drink in addition to what you eat now is going to lose you one single pound of weight.

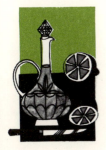

This idea may have arisen partly because people tend to refer to foods which are not normally fattening as "slimming" foods. Lemon juice and vinegar are "slimming" foods in that respect. They certainly won't *add* to your weight.

There is also a belief in circulation that these things can take the edge off your appetite. There's certainly no harm in trying a glass of lemon juice (unsweetened, mind you) before meals to see if it will help you to eat less.

It has been suggested, too, that by taking a glass of unsweetened lemon juice in the morning, and so getting used to "sharper" drinks, you will cease to want sweet drinks. We think that there is quite a lot in this idea. The woman who stops using any sweetening in her tea, for instance, often finds this hard at first, but after a while she finds that she just can't face a sweet cup of tea.

You certainly can quickly acquire a preference for less sweet drinks.

So, yes, these methods can be helpful. But, of course, they are not going to present the entire solution to your basic overweight problem.

Remember this when you are presented with

one of those new "take this and it will make you slim" theories. The first man who can invent a cure in a bottle for excess weight (one which demands no food restriction) will create one of the biggest medical sensations of the century. He will also, probably, end up as one of the world's richest men. So far, he (and his cure) have not been discovered—it is doubtful if they ever will.

SLIMMING PILLS

Almost as nonsensical a theory is the idea that all you need do to lose weight is pop along to the chemist's and buy a nice little box of pills.

Still, it's a nice, optimistic idea. And how very splendid it would be if only it worked.

There are a variety of these so-called "slimming pills" around, sold under a number of proprietary names. What do they actually do for you?

Well, most of them probably work as a laxative, and that is about all. Do laxatives help you to slim? No, they don't. Bowel movement has nothing at all to do with fat reduction.

We won't waste any more time on these "dream pills", but there is another group of "slimming pills" available only by doctor's prescription, which are more worthy of discussion.

These are the appetite-suppressing pills, like Dexedrine and Preludin. Pills of this kind can be used to some extent as a "will-power substitute". They reduce the appetite and so help you to keep to your diet (but it is, of course, the actual dieting which gives the slimming results).

How desirable are these pills? Well, they are a perfectly reasonable aid for the very few women who just can't seem to stick to any diet, however good it is. They provide her with a "crutch". But we must emphasize that it is much, much better to slim without this "crutch" if you possibly can—

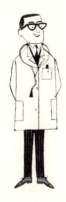

and we genuinely believe that most people can on their correct WOMAN diet.

For one thing, Dexedrine and Preludin may have various side effects which can be undesirable. We must leave it to your doctor to decide how much these will matter to you.

Our concern is the long-term value of diets aided by appetite-suppressing pills compared with diets aided by only a little will-power.

The biggest single virtue of a WOMAN diet based on normal everyday eating is that at the end of it you have got used to eating less of the fattening foods. You will find that you no longer have the desire to eat so much food, especially the food that mainly contributed to your excess weight. You have retrained and readjusted your appestat, you now stand a good chance of *staying* slim.

But if you have dieted with the aid of "a crutch" you are far more likely to go back to your original bad eating habits once the crutch is taken away.

There is, in fact, a third type of pill which might be loosely referred to as "a slimming pill". These pills are those which might be prescribed by a doctor for the woman whose excess weight is caused by glandular problems. Thyroid pills, for instance, come into this category.

They can provide a helpful medical solution to an overweight problem—but, of course, *only* for those women who are overweight because of their glands.

INJECTIONS One of the more modern, pricey and fashionable "methods" of weight reduction owes its prestige to a really smart new angle—injections!

Ah, now here we have something really new and impressive. But does it work?

Well, we must admit that it seems to work, since

39

women who have undergone a series of these hormone injections (the hormones are extracted from the urine of pregnant women) have usually lost weight. Sometimes an impressive amount.

But we are indebted to a group of rather sceptical medical scientists for explaining to us why this method does work.

It is important to know that the women who are given the injection treatment are *also given a slimming diet* to follow.

The medical men who decided to test this method put groups of overweight volunteers on this same diet, and also gave them a course of injections. But what they didn't tell their guinea-pigs was that while some of them were being given the hormone extract injections, others were injected with an equal amount of plain water.

What happened? They all lost weight very well indeed—and the water-injected slimmers lost it just as quickly as the others!

The *diet* was responsible for the weight loss. The injections were responsible only for the confidence that helped them to keep to it.

Remember that the problems so many people find in trying to lose weight lie in their minds, and not in their bodies.

In this book we are hoping to give you the faith and enthusiasm to overcome these problems. We think that you will find this to be the only "injection" of confidence that you need.

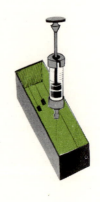

MASSAGE AND MACHINES

By all means enrol for a course of massage during your slimming campaign if you wish to do so. It is stimulating and invigorating. But remember that it is your diet that will lose you the weight.

Massage without dieting is a quite useless method of slimming. The output of energy by

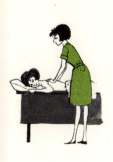

someone else (the masseuse) is not going to use up any of the surplus food that *you* have eaten.

Exercise, and we say this rather sadly because we have our lazy moments too, is a strictly do-it-yourself business. Any amount of pounding and pummelling on your torso by someone else will not do anything at all to remove *your* fat.

However, we often find that women who take a course of massage while they are dieting lose weight particularly well. Their massage obviously helps to make them feel good, and boost their morale.

And these are no small considerations when you are keeping to a diet.

We are going to link up "slimming machines" with massage because their usefulness is along very much the same lines.

A number of slimming salons provide rather pricey courses of treatment based on what more or less amounts to massage by machine. There are, in addition, some rather expensive machines which can be bought for home use.

These machines are usually powered by batteries or electricity, and what they do is produce vibrations. Attachments are put against the fatty pads of the body and they pound away at high speed, giving a not unpleasant sensation.

We have tried them ourselves, and it was great fun. We got the same nice feeling of relaxation that we get when a hairdresser is brushing away at our hair while a manicurist is filing away at our nails (a job we hate anyway).

Watching work—as anyone who has stood around that hole in the road knows—is a tonic. And when the work is being done, by man or machine, on your behalf, it becomes sheer luxury.

It's a nice psychological boost for the slimmer

who may feel she deserves a little pampering, but we must emphasize again that *unless you are dieting at the same time* even the most expensive machines can't help you to lose weight.

METHODS WEIRD AND WONDERFUL

We have covered the most popular non-diet "methods" of slimming in this chapter, but we certainly haven't waded through all the nonsense. It would take the best part of this book to do that. And even if we tried, some other ingenious soul would have thought up some new logic-defying cures for excess weight before our pages were in print!

Just think of some of the things they invent: there are powders you can sprinkle in your bath, waxes that you can paint over your spare tires, rollers, potions and creams.

One of the latest ideas, which we rather treasure, is a "slimming" jam. This jam contains a small percentage of a substance which swells in the body, and tends to reduce your appetite by making you feel full. But to achieve this object in any effective way it would be necessary to devour practically a whole pot of jam in a day. You may eat less of other things. But think what all that jam is going to do to your figure!

Having told you the real facts about slimming, we feel that we can now quite safely leave it to your own good sense to dispose of all these so-called "slimming methods".

Ask yourself these questions:
1. **Have I tried to lose weight by drastically cutting down on all the foods I eat?**
2. **If so, how long did I manage to keep to this type of diet?**

CHAPTER 5
THE DIETS THAT WORK BEST

WE'VE COME TO THE POINT where, having exhausted by now all the other possibilities, there is only one solution left to this problem of overweight. Like it or not, it *must* be a diet.

But the all-important question is, of course: What kind of diet?

Think back for the moment to your basic reason for being overweight: it is that you are eating more food than your body is able to use up. Well, the solution then, surely, must simply be to eat less of everything? If you cut down the portions of all the foods you eat, it seems obvious that you really must lose weight.

This is where we can mention for the first time a word that we have so far very carefully avoided. That word is "calorie". And a calorie is nothing more nor less than just another word for that unit of energy we have been talking about so much.

But we have banned it from previous chapters of this book because in most people's minds it has become inseparably linked with another word—and that is: "counting".

You must have heard of "calorie-counting"! Who hasn't? It's penetrated the consciousness of even your bony elderly uncle, and the first thing he will say if by any chance you should refuse that second helping of pie is:

"Ha ha! Counting your calories, eh?"

Quite honestly, we wish to goodness everyone would now forget that the expression "calorie-counting" ever existed.

The sort of diet we mentioned above—that is, cutting down on the portions of all the food that you eat—is the basis of this calorie-counting method. All foods are listed in accordance with the number of calories that they contain. During the course of any one day you are allowed to eat only a certain total of calories, and must ration out all your food accordingly.

Calorie-counting obviously had something about it that appealed to the public imagination. This method of dieting swept like a whirlwind through both England and America. We even played our own part in it, and introduced a calorie-counting scheme to our readers.

A NEW VIEW

The point we want to make here is that although calorie-counting was the best dieting method then, it isn't the best dieting method *now*. There is now a much easier, more effective and even healthier method of dieting, as you will learn in the chapter you are reading now, the method that we follow in all our diets.

We hope that the writing of this book will once and for all label those calorie-counting diets as being "plain old-fashioned"—and if we manage to do this, then we believe we shall really have achieved something special.

But let us get one thing straight. You will lose weight *only* if you reduce calories. The point is, though, that the up-to-date way does not involve *counting* calories. If you follow our diets, the calories will be reduced without your having to count them. You eat as much as you like of quite a lot of foods, but "as much as you like" ends up by representing fewer calories.

Our "ideal" diet-method, then, is really a way of reducing calories without the mathematical chore of keeping strict account of them. Simple. So simple, in fact, that it has led to an American best-seller called—in type large enough to be almost hysterical—CALORIES DON'T COUNT. Now that is going *too* far . . .

As you will see later, it is quite sensible to say:

"Don't count calories." It is, however, just not true to say: "Calories don't count." The book of that title gave its American readers a lot of fine-sounding talk about metabolism, nutrition, and so on. *In practice*, it works out as our own simple method of dieting.

But we'll graciously admit that the book, extravagant as it is, has perhaps helped the cause in one way: it has given some American ladies the idea that it is possible to lose weight without the need to try and be a genius at arithmetic! And that *is* true.

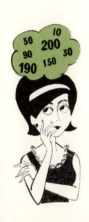

To understand the reasons for calorie-counting no longer being the best method of slimming, and to understand the full virtues of the newer and better method, it is first necessary to have some appreciation of just the simplest, basic facts about the functions of food.

WHAT FOOD DOES FOR YOU

So far, for the sake of simplicity, we have been talking about food as no more than the essential fuel for our supply of energy. You may well have got the impression that all food is either used up in energy, or stored as fat.

However, that is far from being the full story. Food is necessary for other purposes. Our bodies, in many ways, are just like machines. Anyone who has owned a car (and grumbled at the cost of spare parts) will readily appreciate that engines just don't go on forever. They will gradually wear away and they need regular repair or, from time to time, actual replacement.

In the same way our bodies need gradually to repair and replace worn tissue. And they find the components necessary for this from some of the foods we eat.

A car needs oil regularly as well. And in the

same way, our bodies need to have other essential nutrients just to keep everything ticking over smoothly and efficiently.

What are the nutrients essential for the basic functions of our bodies? And from what foods do we get them?

THE VITAL NUTRIENTS

Among the very first essentials for basic body tissue repair are some substances that are called amino-acids. These substances are supplied by the protein in our food.

Now protein, like most other essential elements, is found in a wide variety of foods—including bread and green vegetables. But the proteins with the amino-acids that we most need are found in their highest concentration in animal foods, like meat, fish, milk, cheese and eggs.

These foods, in fact, are the ones that we generally refer to as "the proteins".

They are, as we indicated above, a first essential in any healthy diet.

Another group of nutrients that are absolutely essential to the functions of the body are the mineral elements. It is these which supply the raw materials needed for blood, bones and teeth, and also the necessary salt content of our bodies. There are a great number of different mineral elements occurring in minute quantities in a great number of foods. It is most unlikely that any person would go short of the majority of them, whatever her diet might be.

However, there are three important ones that could possibly be deficient in some of the more ill-designed of the crash diets. These are calcium, iron and iodine.

Again, we must stress that these elements are present to some degree in many foods. But they are found chiefly in milk and cheese (*calcium*), meat, green vegetables and eggs (*iron*), and fish and other sea foods (*iodine*).

The third group of these essential nutrients have probably been brought to your attention already by health-and-fitness enthusiasts. For this group consists of the vitamins. And they are, roughly speaking, the chemical compounds necessary to keep the body "ticking over nicely". We can think of them working for us just as the oil works for the motor car we talked about.

Vitamins are essentially an IN-thing in the age that we live in. Their importance has been quite rightly recognized. But many impressionable people seem to have gone a little overboard on the idea of vitamin-packed living.

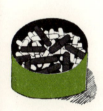

We read about the visiting American film stars who take about fifty pills a day, and attribute to them their vitality and their youthfulness. Industries at home have set out to convince people that they *must* have vitamin pills to be healthy. There even exists what almost amounts to a "vitamins by H.P." scheme.

So, while we are stressing the importance of those vitamins, we would nevertheless like to take this opportunity to get the whole thing a little more in proportion.

The facts are these: If you eat a well-balanced diet you are almost certainly getting all the vitamins that you require. And your body just does not use more vitamins than it needs. So all the concentration of vitamins in those precious pills is very often being disposed of as waste.

However, bear in mind that vitamins which are prescribed by a doctor where for some special reason there is a deficiency are a completely different matter. Our scepticism extends only to haphazard buying of vitamin pills by a normal healthy person on a normal healthy diet.

What must this normal healthy diet include to supply the correct amount of vital vitamins? Let's consider the four most essential:

Vitamin A: which helps keep smooth the skin, eyes and soft lining tissue of the body, is found mainly in the fat of milk (also butter and cheese) and is added to margarine.

There is an even higher concentration in liver, especially fish livers and in cod liver oil and halibut oil. Vitamin A is also found in green vegetables, and yellow and orange ones (swedes, carrots etc.) though in a different form.

B Group Vitamins: which are necessary for many functions of the body are found in various amounts in most foods—but especially in animal foods (and, in particular, meat, liver, milk). Most of them are also found in cereals.

Vitamin C: which is particularly important for a healthy skin is probably the best known and the most "popular" of all the vitamins. It is found for the most part in fruits and in vegetables, particularly in oranges, blackcurrants, strawberries and in the green vegetables.

Vitamin D: which plays such a part in the bone formation of growing children, is absent in many foods, but it is found in butter and margarine, in animal and fish livers and their oils.

While we are summing up this necessarily brief and simple account of the essential nutrients, it is important to stress that they really are *vital*. It would take pages to tell of all the illnesses that can be the result of a severe deficiency in any of them. However, there is no need to get obsessed with the idea, and start measuring out nutrients instead of planning proper meals. As long as you are living on a well-varied menu of everyday foods, your body will be well supplied with the nutrients it requires and can safely be left to look after itself without your having to worry about it.

And now—back to the subject of slimming!

THE SNAGS OF CALORIE-COUNTING

If we think back to our calorie-counting dieter we can assume, from what we have just learned, that her diet may be fairly safe. She's probably reducing the size of the portions of the food she eats, and not necessarily limiting the variety of it. And as a good variety in the foods you eat is the important safety factor, because small amounts at least of the vital nutrients are found in so many foods, we won't complain of these calorie-counting diets on that score.

What, then, is the problem the calorie-counter has to face?

Purely and simply, it is just that she usually feels jolly hungry!

In order to lose weight on this type of diet she will usually find herself having to cut down pretty drastically the foods that she normally finds are satisfying to her.

Now this is all very well for people who are really strong-willed.

But how many of us can claim in all honesty that we are strong-willed enough to go really hungry for a few months? You will remember that one of the main reasons for the failure of any diet is that it makes too great a demand on our very often limited store of will-power.

Until only a few years ago, all diets did tend

to ask rather too much of our self-restraint, and all we could do was grimly to grit our teeth and try to make the best of them.

Nowadays, thank goodness, that cast-iron will-power is no longer necessary.

MEDICAL DISCOVERIES

Since excess weight became recognized as the health danger—and even killer—that it is, medical scientists have been constantly experimenting to find new and better ways of reducing it.

Of course, experiments had been going on in a haphazard sort of way for many years before. And in fact, almost a hundred years ago, there was one doctor who produced a theory that came very close indeed to the best present-day method of weight reduction.

But after thorough scientific exploration modern experts have been able to confirm this:

Weight reduction need not demand the cutting down of all types of food. Usually, it is much more easily and effectively achieved by the deliberate restriction of just one group of foods.

To understand this, we must divide most of the basic foods we eat into three groups:

The protein-rich foods: animal foods like meat, fish, cheese and eggs.

The fats: butter, margarine and cooking fats (also so-called "invisible fats" contained in many foods, including milk and cheese, the lean parts of meat, fish, and chocolate).

The carbohydrate-rich foods: cereal-based foods of which flour is the most popular, rice, spaghetti and certain root vegetables like potatoes. In addition—and most important—sugar!

By firmly curtailing the foods in just any one of

these three groups, while eating quite normally from the other two groups, you *could* manage to lose your excess weight.

This obviously represents a big step forward from the old-fashioned "cut down on everything" school of thought. But we must consider very carefully which particular group it is that we are going to choose to restrict.

CAN PROTEINS BE LIMITED?

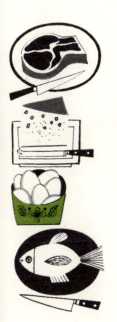

We'll take the proteins first. American medical scientists have proved, in tests on overweight people, that a low protein diet can work. But the scientists concerned were quick to express their doubts about the safety of such diets, unless conducted under the closest medical supervision.

Take a look back at the sections on medical discoveries and vital nutrients and you'll see why. You can't fail to notice the importance of proteins, how often the protein-rich foods are mentioned. The body relies on them much more for the repair of tissue, than for the creation of body fat.

Nutritionists strongly advise that we should take in a good supply of protein foods every day.

To slim by drastically curtailing proteins would be to deprive our bodies of necessities. And if we persisted we would almost certainly become ill.

There's another point to be considered too. Some foods supply a larger amount of energy units—or calories, as we can now safely call them —than others. And you will remember that it is this excessive intake of energy units that becomes converted to fat.

Of the three groups, the proteins in our eating give us the lowest number of calories. They are generally more concerned with bodily repair than the generating of energy.

So if we were to eat normally from the other

high-calorie foods, we really would have to curb proteins drastically in order to lose weight, and this would be slimming the hard way. It would also demand much calculating and counting out of very exact portions.

A specifically low-protein diet would be much more difficult to keep to than the method of calorie-counting we have already mentioned, which makes you cut down on all foods.

Therefore, on health grounds and on practical grounds we can—and *must*—dismiss the method of restricting protein alone as a safe and wise way of slimming.

HOW MUCH DO WE NEED FATS?

On to the second group then. The limiting of fats would seem to suggest itself as the obvious answer to many people. We know some foods are higher in calories than others. And fats are certainly among the high-calorie foods.

But let's see what would actually happen if you tried to follow a low-fat diet.

To begin with, it must be realized that the foods that we normally think of as fats make up only about half of our daily consumption of fats. There are, if you remember, those "invisible fats" which are found in many other foods, so it wouldn't just be a matter of eating dry bread and of throwing out the frying pan.

An even more important fact is this: fats have a high satiety value. Those we include in a meal tend to make the food go through our stomach more slowly than they otherwise would.

And that means that we are satisfied for longer or, if you like to put it this way, it means we are hungry again less quickly.

So any diet short in fats would have a very low satiety value. In fact, for most of the time we

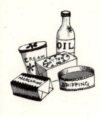

would find ourselves hungry, and also, as has been discovered from experience, irritable, tired and depressed.

Obviously, the low-fat diet which produces these results is far from being the ideal easy diet that we are looking for. It would be very hard to keep to. But before we dismiss the subject of fats entirely we will mention one dieting theory about them which gained considerable publicity both in America and in this country a few years ago.

Some medical men, on the track of the truth that reduction of fats is not actually the good slimming method that it was once thought to be, pretty well went the full circle. They then decided that not only did fats not make you fat—they actually made you slim!

Their suggestion was all based on the idea that certain fats increased the metabolic (food-using) rate of the body, and so burned up other foods, which might otherwise have been converted to body fat. So, following this line of "reasoning", they advocated diets containing a very high amount of certain fats for this purpose.

In the absence of any really convincing evidence to support this theory we prefer to take the view of Professor John Yudkin, with his unparalleled reputation in the field of dieting research in Britain. To put it bluntly, Professor Yudkin believes that this theory of the slimming value of fat is "rather a lot of nonsense".

As he explains it quite clearly: "When the sole reason for gaining weight is over-eating, how can you possibly lose weight by *adding* anything to what you eat!"

In the diets that we shall be telling you about, which you'll find in Part II, you will be free to eat what fat you like, but will probably find that you

53

are eating a little less than usual because of the restriction of other foods which are so often eaten along with fats.

CARBOHYDRATE REDUCTION

Now we come to the only method that is left to us —the limiting of carbohydrates. And this time we have struck gold!

There are several sound reasons a low carbohydrate diet works well, and works safely.

It works well because carbohydrate foods are high suppliers of calories (or energy units). They contain lots of calories but often little in the way of proteins, minerals or vitamins. More than other foods, they usually account for much of the excess energy we store up as fat.

To see how safely it works you can check back to the vital nutrient section again.

The carbohydrate foods are not mentioned often. This does not mean that carbohydrates are useless foods and contain none of the essential nutrients we need, for they contain many of them, but mostly in small amounts.

However, in almost every case—and this is the essential point—all these nutrients can be supplied equally well by the protein and fat foods found in our diet.

The carbohydrate foods are mainly what we might term "the artificial foods"—that is, the foods that we managed largely to do without in our primitive state. They also tend to be the foods we eat in bulk in the present day.

If we are going to follow a diet which is based on the cutting down of carbohydrates only, how does that work out in practice?

Well, to begin with, without making any efforts to do so, we tend automatically to limit, to some extent, our intake of fats. Less bread means, of course, less butter. And just think of all the fat that goes into pastry—that will be cut out, too. There will be less potato mashed with butter, fewer fried potatoes . . .

We're not going to limit drastically our intake of fats (even though they are high in calories) because that would make us feel too hungry to be able to keep to our diets successfully. But the slight automatic reduction is going to help a little, while the carbohydrate-cutting does the major part of the slimming job.

What about protein foods? Well, we shall probably increase their intake a little since, along with the carbohydrate-free vegetables that we shall still eat freely, they are going to be the mainstay of our diet.

But proteins, if you remember, on the whole are a great deal more concerned with bodily repair than with the mere production of energy. They are low in calories.

They can, however, still provide us with much of the energy we need for our daily activities—when we combine them with the fats and the small ration of carbohydrate that we allow in our diets. And remember, on a diet we want to encourage the body to draw on those fatty stores of energy that have been laid up.

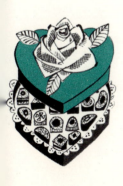

Remember, also, that the carbohydrates, and particularly the sweet foods, tend to be the basis of our "just for pleasure" eating. Since chocolates, ice-creams and cakes are rarely eaten simply to satisfy any real hunger, for the most part they supply only "excess" energy, (which we want to avoid!) when our normal meals have provided all the energy we can use up.

So carbohydrate reduction automatically will limit the amount of food we eat, while still allowing us to eat enough of additional things to appease real hunger.

We are not saying that a low carbohydrate diet is the *only* one that can slim you. But what we are saying is that it is the *easiest and safest* of the modern methods—and the one, therefore, that is the most likely to succeed.

It is easier than "calorie-counting" (that is the cutting down on everything) because it generally allows you to eat more food, and have much more freedom in eating.

It is much easier than a low-fat diet since it leaves you feeling much more satisfied, and demands a lot less will-power.

It is much, much safer than a low-protein diet which is very difficult and, as we have explained, can be downright dangerous.

So there we have it. The best of modern methods, and the basis of all the diets that you will find in this book.

Having told you the reasons for our belief that the low-carbohydrate diet is the best one yet invented, we are now going to tell you about some other slimming diets. We'll explain how they could work—and why, in actual practice, they more often than not *don't* work.

First ask yourself these questions:

1. **Just how many bananas could I face in any one day?**
2. **Have I ever managed to keep to a diet which demanded the repeated eating of just one or two foods?**

CHAPTER 6
THE "FAD" DIETS

SO FAR, we hope that you have found this book sensible rather than sensational. But now we are going to give you a surprise, and present you with a diet that ought to make even the most ardent gimmick enthusiast turn pale.

Coffee and doughnuts: that's the complete menu for our new, never-before-discovered diet. The sheer originality should leave you gasping. And, what's more, if you can keep to a diet of nothing but coffee and doughnuts, we can assure you that you will lose weight.

However, we think you will have been smart enough to work out that either there must be a snag, or that we must have gone insane.

There is a snag. And you'll find the clue in that phrase "*if you can keep to a diet* of nothing but coffee and doughnuts".

Certainly you would lose weight if you had doughnuts and coffee alone, because there is a limit to the number of doughnuts that even the greatest doughnut-lover can face in one day. Out of sheer revulsion you would drastically cut down your eating (and automatically, your calorie intake, too) very swiftly.

After eating doughnut after doughnut on Monday and Tuesday, you'd notice you were eating fewer doughnuts on Wednesday and Thursday, fewer still on Friday. By Saturday, death itself would seem preferable to a doughnut.

Of course, our doughnut diet is all a lot of nonsense, but it does illustrate very well how some of the famous "fad" diets could work, and why, in actual practice, they *don't*.

BANANAS AND MILK

The banana-and-milk diet is among the best known of these slimming methods. But the facts and the failures behind this diet apply equally well

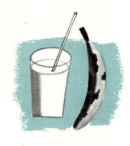

to any other diets which limit your eating to just one or two specific foods.

The banana-and-milk diet is nutritionally more sound than our own coffee-and-doughnut diet—which we thought up only five minutes before we wrote it down. In fact, you would be able to sustain life for quite a long time on bananas and milk, mainly because the two combined contain most of the nutrients essential to health. But how long could you face it?

Bananas can become just as big a bore as our doughnuts. And if they were the only choice of food allowed you would definitely cut down on your calorie intake.

But the fact is, unless you possess a will of iron, you just can't continue this monotonous pattern of eating for very long.

The diet won't work for the simple reason that you won't be able to keep to it.

As our nutritional adviser once remarked:

"If there is any woman who has managed to keep to a diet of bananas and milk for over a month, I would be delighted to meet her and shake her by the hand!"

FRUIT AND VEGETABLE DIETS

Diets which limit your food to fruits only, or to fruit and vegetables only, come in very much the same category as banana-and-milk diets—but they provide a little more variety.

Again, they work very much on the principle that you will not want to eat too much of any one particular type of food, and so you will take in fewer calories than usual.

We have no quarrel with these diets as short-term diets—and that is how they are usually presented. Beauty farms often put their clients on this type of diet for a couple of days, and some people make a habit of eating only fruit and vegetables for a day or two every month.

We, ourselves, include some days of mainly fruit and vegetable eating in two of the diets we have designed in the second part of the book.

But it would be silly to consider a diet of fruit and vegetables alone as a long-term diet, designed to pare away a stone or two. For one thing, it would not be nutritionally sound. And, just like the banana-and-milk diet, it would sorely tax your will-power through sheer monotony.

We have come across some diets—"Clock-watchers" we call them—which suggest that you starve during part of the day, then have a good old pig at a certain time. One of our dieters, much to our surprise, presented us with a diet she'd been given by her doctor, based on this idea.

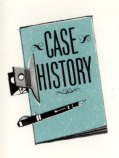

The poor girl—Sheila, she was called—came to see us because she had discovered that she "couldn't slim on a diet".

We asked to look at the diet she had been trying to follow, and saw that she had been asked to live on little more than the odd lettuce leaf and apple until six o'clock every evening. After six o'clock, she was told, she could eat as much as she liked of whatever she liked.

Obviously, the idea was that she would eat less over a limited time, from six o'clock onwards, than she would during a whole day.

We think the good doctor sadly under-estimated the number of calories that a healthy girl can pack away at one go. The evening meal that the ravenous Sheila usually tackled was quite impressive. And she didn't lose weight.

Not only did this diet lack effective results, it

59

also demanded that Sheila should put up with a lengthy period of hunger each day. And we don't believe that there are very many people who can voluntarily stay hungry for long.

Of course you could get used to eating virtually just one big meal in a day. But it would take a considerable time to become accustomed to it.

We felt sure that Sheila would find dieting much easier if she could spread out her calorie intake through the day. So we gave her one of our diets which allowed three balanced meals.

"I didn't know that dieting could be as easy as this," she told us.

We explained that with most people, the easier the diet, the more sure the results—we could never see any point in creating added difficulties.

Sheila proved our point by losing weight steadily and well—and staying right with her diet until she had achieved her object.

Incidentally, many people have the impression that meals they eat at night are going to be more fattening than earlier meals, because they are using up little energy afterwards. But it makes no difference at what time of the day you eat your calories. You could use the evening ones up on the following morning!

The total intake of food and the total usage of energy over the whole period of twenty-four hours is the real factor to consider.

SWEDISH MILK DIETS

The well-known Swedish milk diets work on even tougher stop-go tactics. The basis of these diets is that for three or four days a week you take nothing but four glasses of milk with a special formula added. On the days in-between you have a more or less normal diet.

Well, perhaps our readership is just lacking in

super-women—but we haven't come across many steely characters who could get through three or four days each week without solid food.

Realizing that firm resolution is much easier to sustain for one day than a whole week, we use the "stop-go" tactic to a small extent in our "Flying Starters" diets (beginning on page 159). These two diets are recommended to the strongest-willed of our readers only—but even then they don't call for more than a fraction of the self-restraint that is demanded by the Swedish milk diets.

Our own belief is that many people start off on these Swedish milk diets, but few, except those who have only a few pounds to lose, can manage to complete the course. We take our hats off to you if you have succeeded in doing so.

They are far too tough for us.

DRINKING MAN'S DIET

There are some new diets that tend to attract devotees for no greater reason than that they sound so revolutionary and remarkable. And as long as they work we are all for them.

We make our own diets attractive and appealing in every possible way because we know that if we have attracted your enthusiasm and confidence we have got you off to a good start.

The Drinking Man's diet is just one of these revolutionary-sounding methods of slimming. It came over from America, and has been met with some enthusiasm on both sides of the Atlantic during the past year or two.

The Drinking Man's diet sounds splendidly human and jolly. And what's more it seems to dispose firmly of rotten old kill-joys like ourselves who say: "Cut out the alcohol" on a diet.

As a matter of fact, the Drinking Man's Diet is based fundamentally on the soundest slimming method that we know of—the low-carbohydrate we use in our own WOMAN diets.

Slimmers are first of all taught how to follow the low-carbohydrate method of dieting, and then they are told that they should drink their normal amount of alcohol—*but no more*.

Of course, they lose weight because of their food restriction. They would naturally lose weight more rapidly if they cut out their alcohol, too—but as long as they are happy, and slimming, we would be the last to grumble.

In our own dieting method, we believe that speed is important. A woman loses faith and enthusiasm unless she is rewarded by fairly fast results. And as alcohol has a high carbohydrate-equivalent it has to be largely sacrificed to speed.

However, if you find it hard to give up alcohol for a period, and aren't too worried about speed, you could make your own "drinking girl's diet" by taking your normal amount of alcohol, and following one of the faster diets in this book.

CRASH DIETS

What exactly is a "crash diet"? Well, it's a loose sort of term that is usually applied to a diet that allows the very minimum amount of food and calls for the very maximum amount of will-power. Top speed slimming is the aim, and we have no quarrel with this—with certain reservations.

On a crash diet you might miss out certain meals altogether. Your aim would be to accept and come to terms with hunger, and to eat the very minimum amount of food in a day.

Crash diets are rarely advocated by magazines these days. But we quite often come across women who have attempted to put themselves on a "do-it-yourself" version.

Quite honestly, we don't worry too much about

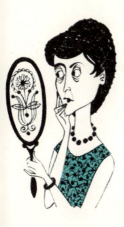

these diets—because they are usually abandoned before they can do any harm.

But the question arises: Is it possible to try and slim too quickly?

We believe that it is, because a diet that is too drastically limited in food is very often short in essential nutrients, as well.

One of the first things our would-be dieters nearly always say to us is:

"I don't want to end up looking all haggard. Are you sure this won't happen?"

We can assure them that it won't happen on our diets. Even when women have lost a considerable amount of weight around the face and chin we have never found that they looked pinched, drawn or droopy. On the contrary, they have begun to look younger, firmer, more attractive.

But on a real crash diet you *would* begin to look haggard. A body that is being starved of essential nutrients will not lose just fat. Muscles and other parts of the body will suffer too.

The high speed diets in this book are designed to allow a little margin of safety. But we wouldn't advise anything much faster, if you're really aiming to improve your looks, and health.

THOUSANDS OF DIETS

In concluding this chapter we will point out a fact that you have probably appreciated already.

It isn't difficult to invent a diet that *could* work. We could probably invent one a day for the next five years without any difficulty.

But it is much more difficult to invent a diet that *will* work in practice.

Diets—including most of those we have mentioned in this chapter—rarely fail. But *slimmers* often fail because they can't keep to a diet.

We have this fact very much in mind when we

63

design our own diets for you. And we put great importance on another factor, too.

There isn't much point in losing 2 stone in three months if you put it back again as quickly. That is why we base our diets as closely as possible on normal everyday eating.

The failing of most "fad" diets is that they are of little use in re-training the appestat.. When you have finished with them there is nothing to stop your going back to eating in exactly the same way as you did before you started dieting.

But when you have succeeded with a WOMAN diet, you have become used to a pattern of eating that can now become a basis of everyday eating.

We won't say that you will never be able to look a cream bun in the face again. But carbohydrates are likely to take a smaller place on your menu from now on. You have acquired a good habit that will help you to keep slim.

Now ask yourself these questions:
   1. **Have I ever tried slimming with the aid of branded slimming foods?**
   2. **If so, how much did they help me?**

CHAPTER 7
BRANDED SLIMMING FOODS

LIQUID DIETS

BESIDES THE DIETS we mentioned in the previous chapter there are a number which are based on the use of branded slimming foods. Since these are widely advertised, and therefore well known, we feel that they deserve some discussion.

Just how much help can they be?

Well, we'll consider first the meal-substitute liquid diets—like Complan. This can be used as a total diet for swift weight loss, or as a replacement for one or two meals daily.

Originally, Complan was designed to provide nourishment for those unconscious or seriously ill in hospital. It is still used widely in hospitals and in homes for providing a nourishing food supplement for patients of all kinds. But it is recommended now also for slimmers.

By taking a measured amount each day of one of these products you can be sure of taking a measured amount of calories. So they certainly provide an exact diet—more exact than our own, in fact, which allow you to give or take a few calories to make life easier.

As the basis of any major slimming campaign, however, these products fall down for many of the same reasons as the "fad" diets.

It takes a strong will to abandon not only all the foods you like, but also all the foods that you normally eat, even for a limited period. A diet of liquid and nothing else is bound to be monotonous. At the end of it you have not been re-schooled in normal eating habits, so there is nothing to prevent you from going back to the way of eating that made you fat.

However, for a slower diet these products are also suggested as a substitute for just one or two meals of the day—or else as a total diet on

65

selected days of the week.

This would be a very much easier routine, but because of the temptation to eat more food at the normal meals, it would probably turn out to be a very slow one.

There is no doubt that these diets can work when the will is very strong indeed. And, of course, they are completely trouble-free, with no extra shopping—and no cooking at all.

But however hard we struggle to be fair, when we compare them with our own methods, on the joint grounds of ease and effectiveness, we can't but feel that they present a very hard and hazardous path to slimming success.

SLIMMING BISCUITS

Slimming biscuits like Limmits Crackers, Limmits Chocolate Wholemeal Biscuits, Trimmets Wafers, Trimmets Break, Bisks Sandwich Biscuits, Bisks Milk Chocolate Biscuits and Simbix Diet Biscuits are designed to replace one or more meals each day.

They are well balanced nutritionally, and are also designed to act as complete calorie-controlled meals. If taken to replace normal meals, with a pint of milk daily, they will form a calorie-controlled diet.

The flavours of these biscuits are varied and attractive, and this would certainly be a fast and effective method of losing weight. But we do feel that a complete diet of slimming biscuits is only for the extremely strong-willed. It must get monotonous over a sustained period of time, and certainly demands more will-power than any of the diets in this book.

These products, however, have certain practical advantages for the busy slimmer. They are easy to carry to the office, and certainly win hands down on the washing-up! But to achieve results of any speed this procedure would have to be combined with a plan of calorie-controlled meals for the remainder of the day.

Most of these biscuits also contain a product called methyl-cellulose which we describe in the next section. It helps them to be more "filling".

A group of other products, Boots Diet Milk Chocolate, Limmits Soup and Limmits Chocolate, come into the same category as the biscuits. They are designed as complete meal replacements (preferably for just one or two meals a day). Don't make the mistake of eating them in addition to normal meals!

APPETITE REDUCERS

There is another type of branded slimming aid totally different from the others we have discussed in this chapter. We are thinking of products like Pastils 808, Slim Disks, Intrim Golden Grains, Trihextin Capsules, and Q 70.

These products are not food substitutes. They are meant to be taken at a prescribed time (usually fifteen to twenty minutes) before a meal, with the object of making you feel less hungry—and helping you to keep to your diet.

All these products, whether they are capsules, pastilles, biscuits, or powders to be made up into a drink, contain harmless substances (methyl-cellulose or vegetable ingredients) which just swell up your tummy to give a comfortably full feeling. Our medical advisers are quite happy about methyl-cellulose because it has no side-effects and is not habit forming.

Products of this kind can be helpful to people who find difficulty in keeping to a diet—but it is the diet, remember, which slims you.

Another well-known product, Ayds, also comes

into the group of appetite reducers, but works on an entirely different principle. Ayds are rather like small caramels and contain liquid glucose, vitamins and minerals. Their main object is to raise the blood-sugar level very quickly (glucose is swiftly absorbed into the blood), because it is only when your blood-sugar level is low that you feel really hungry.

To help suppress your appetite at the strategic time they should be taken about 20 minutes before a meal, preferably with a hot drink. As they contain glucose they do, of course, have a carbohydrate value of their own, but not enough to interfere with a reasonably swift diet if taken as prescribed. Each Ayds cube contains approximately 30 calories.

The only thing against appetite reducers is that after you stop taking them at the end of the diet you are more likely to go back to eating larger amounts of food. You haven't retrained your appetite quite as well as you would have by relying on your diet and will-power alone.

However it is very much better to diet with these aids than not to diet at all. So try relying on our kindly diets and a little will-power first, and turn to this extra assistance if will-power fails you.

BACK TO CARBO-HYDRATES

Having discussed many of the other methods of dieting, we believe that you, like us, will be all the more convinced that the low-carbohydrate diet, based on everyday foods, really takes some beating for ease and effectiveness.

So ask yourself these questions:

1. **Is my dieting will-power strong, average, weak or variable?**

2. **What factors count most to me in making a diet easy to follow?**

CHAPTER 8

THE DIET THAT'S RIGHT FOR YOU

NOW YOU KNOW practically all you need to know about truly effective slimming methods. This is where the action starts.

In this chapter you will find the guide to your own ideal WOMAN diet. There are ten of them at the end of this book—each one based on the sound medical principles that we have explored together.

Why so many? Well, let us make clear at the beginning that as far as your *body* is concerned every one of these diets can work for you. Each one, if carefully followed, is a guaranteed weight shedder for every healthy woman.

But in planning diets, and studying them in action for many years, WOMAN experts have discovered that the body is only one factor to be taken into consideration when choosing a diet to suit an individual.

There are other even more important factors to consider. In particular, the will-power and the way of life of the woman concerned.

The diet that doesn't work is the one that isn't followed. And if you choose one that demands too much of your will-power, or becomes really hard work because it simply doesn't fit into your way of life, you can guess what happens. You can probably prove what happens from your own past experience.

That is why we think it most important to guide you to the one diet that is exactly right for you as an individual.

If you flip through the back pages now you will see that the diets are divided into four sections. There are the "Diets That Let You Choose", the "Flying-Starters" and the "Food-Lovers' Diets" and the diets that are "Swift-and-Straightforward". In addition there is one special after-pregnancy diet provided. And so, unless you have quite recently had a baby, in which case the choice is obvious, the problem now is to decide in which section lies that diet which was just made for you. Here are some questions which will solve it for you:

WHERE CHOICE
MATTERS MOST

Ask yourself these questions:

Is this you? A housewife with a whole family's appetites to cook for as well as yourself. A girl with definite likes and dislikes about food.

Are these your diet problems? You find it difficult to stick to a set menu if all the family has to be considered when you are making plans for a meal. It is hard for you to eat what you are told, and often you don't like the food suggested.

Then your perfect diet is in the "Diets That Let You Choose" section.

The WOMAN diets in this section have been specially devised to give CHOICE. Two of them, in fact, allow you to eat practically anything you fancy, within the bounds of weight reduction. And could anything be nicer than managing to slim on your own favourite foods!

Slimmers who put choice and variety first will clearly see the futility of fad diets like bananas-and-milk, which were referred to earlier in this book, when they contrast them with the freedom allowed in the diets in this section.

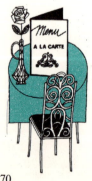

The housewife on a WOMAN free-choice diet has no need to eat alone or prepare special meals. She can use her diet as the basis of economical and popular family meals. Members of the family with no weight worries can have additional helpings of potatoes, pudding, and other carbo-hydrate foods.

If you answered a firm "Yes" to the questions

above, look for the symbol of the menu by the diets at the end of the book. But if these questions didn't seem to get right to the root of your own problem, perhaps the next ones will.

WHERE A FLYING START PAYS DIVIDENDS

Is this you? A single girl who cooks for herself, or a housewife who is keen enough on losing weight to follow quite a different eating pattern from the rest of the family. Essentially an enthusiast, raring to go on a diet, willing (at this moment) to starve, if necessary, to get slim.

Is this your diet problem? Unfortunately that initial enthusiasm rarely lasts. For perhaps a couple of days at a time you can be really tough with yourself. But then . . . The strict diets that really appeal to you usually go overboard after you've been on them only a few days.

Then your perfect diet is in the "Flying-Starters" section.

The WOMAN diets in this section are designed to make full use of those short bursts of enthusiasm of which you are capable. Then, just when your will-power is sagging, they provide the necessary boost by changing and easing the pace.

These diets differ in one essential way from most other WOMAN diets. We always stress the importance of balanced eating; and the correct amount of health-giving proteins, minerals and fats are normally measured out and allocated on our menus day by day.

However, our medical advisers have shown that for the purposes of dieting it is not always necessary to consider food balance on a *daily* basis—as long as it is being achieved over a short period of time.

We have made full use of this fact in these "flying start" diets. For a couple of days you may find yourself on practically nothing but liquids, or proteins, or on fruit and vegetables. But during the course of a week you will be taking in all the food elements necessary for perfect health.

Like all our diets, the "Flying Starters" are perfectly safe for a healthy person. But particularly to slimmers choosing these diets, we would stress the importance of checking with a doctor first if your state of health leaves any room for doubt.

A complete change of eating pattern from day to day has proved to be a definite plus factor in speeding weight reduction. So if speed is your aim, and you answered a firm "Yes" to the questions above, look for the symbol of the runner by the diets at the end of the book. If, however, this slimming method seems to be asking a little too much of your will-power and enthusiasm, you will probably find yourself more ideally reflected in the next questions.

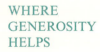

WHERE GENEROSITY HELPS

Is this you? A teenager who frankly loves her food. A housewife who enjoys preparing large and satisfying meals. A hearty eater.

Is this your diet problem? However much you try to stick to "the right" diet foods, sometimes you find yourself just longing for fish and chips or apple dumplings.

Then your perfect diet is in the "Food-Lovers' Diets" section.

The WOMAN diets in this section are different in that you will find among their menus surprising things like porridge, potatoes, meringues—yes, fish and chips and apple dumplings too!

Because they have been expertly balanced with the rest of your planned meals these items can be eaten from time to time without adding on weight. In short, we have taken into account the fact that you are subject to eating temptation (as, indeed, so many people are) and we have allowed you to succumb to it a little *without interfering with your regular weight loss.*

The "Food-Lovers'" diets are particularly tasty and generous. You may even find that the substantial meals seem rather more generous than the ones you are already eating. Of course successful dieting depends on how much you eat. But this can best be adjusted automatically by *what* you eat. And even when you take those "special treats" into account, the diets will firmly curb your intake of carbohydrates.

We would particularly recommend the first diet in this section for the young teenager with a "puppy fat" problem. As long as she is in perfect, normal health, her parents need have none of the old worries on the score of "safety".

It would be no extravagance to claim that WOMAN's "Food-Lovers'" diets stand out as the easiest and safest among all known *effective* methods of slimming. Look for the symbol of the well-filled plate to identify them at the back of the book. But if high speed slimming is more in your line, ask yourself the next questions.

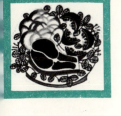

WHERE SPEED LINKS WITH SIMPLICITY

Is this you? A busy housewife with a time limit —you quickly need a new slim figure for a certain special big occasion. A busy career girl with just a few pounds to shed, and a "lets get it over with quick" approach to the situation. **Are these your diet problems?** Most swift diets demand too much fuss, or too much change from normal family eating. You could follow one only if it involved hardly any extra shopping or cooking (no calculations even) and would fit in with family or restaurant eating.

Then your perfect diet is in the "Swift-And-Straightforward Diets" section.

The WOMAN diets in this section are based on normal everyday meals—but with carbohydrates trimmed firmly away so that the weight loss pace is fast.

The meals are all worked out for you, to save time and trouble. They could easily be used as the basis of a family menu (other members of the family adding extra helping of carbohydrate foods). And the career girl who often eats in restaurants would have no difficulty in obtaining diet meals there—particularly if she chooses the diet from this section which allows a certain amount of choice.

If you answered "Yes" to the questions above, look for the symbol of the arrow by the diets at the end of the book, to identify the ones that are right for you.

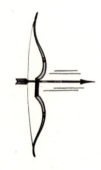

SETTING THE SPEED

The questions above lead you to the right section of diets; when you turn to it you'll see more questions, to pinpoint *the one* diet to suit you in every possible way.

You will also see that *each* diet is given a weight-loss speed rating. This will give you a clear indication of what it demands in will-power. But at this stage you are probably even more keen to know what it means in actual pounds lost each week.

It would be impossible for us to give an exact answer. Individual weight loss patterns vary enormously for many reasons.

Often we find, for instance, that a woman used to a very large amount of sweet and starchy food

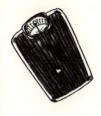

will show a much more sensational weight loss, particularly at the beginning of her diet, than another woman on the same diet who has previously been eating less.

Then, week-to-week weight loss varies too. The first week is usually a cracker. We have known women, usually in the 2 stone-plus overweight group who have lost up to 8 lb. in only seven days (although 4 lb. to 5 lb. would be more usual).

This sudden spurt is caused by the fact that very many overweight bodies have an excessive amount of water tucked away in the tissues.

You remember that ordinarily the amount of water in our bodies is pretty constant. But during a diet we are changing our metabolic (food-using) pattern, and this may alter, for a short time, the way in which we balance our body water.

We may lose more water than usual at first, particularly with the cut in carbohydrates. Or, alternatively, we may retain more water than usual during part of the diet.

The days just before and during the monthly period are particularly affected by this liquid variation.

Frequently we'll find that just before the period a disappointed slimmer will record no weight loss at all on the scales. But just after the period she will record a much greater weight loss than usual. She is delighted—but wonders why.

She has, in fact, been losing *basic* weight steadily all the time. But because the body tends to store a larger amount of liquid than usual just before and during the monthly period she weighs more at that time.

However, having explained why we can't give the exact speed of weight loss on each diet we now give *a very rough "average" estimate* based on our dieting trials.

Average speed loss: An average of 1 lb. a week, very possibly more.

Average-quick speed loss: An average of 2 lb. a week, possibly more.

High speed loss: An average of 3 lb. a week, occasionally more, or a fraction less.

Now ask yourself a few more questions:
1. **Am I quite sure that I'm in perfect health?**
2. **Do I know which are the least fattening sugar substitutes and slimming breads,** or do I just assume that they are all the same?
3. **Have I tried to slim by missing meals**—and did it work?

CHAPTER 9

THE RULES AND THEIR REASONS

RULES ARE SOMETHING the majority of us tend to be bored by, or against.

They are also, according to manufacturers who issue a list of rules (or "instructions") with their products, something that the average British woman seldom bothers to read.

Now you've got us worried there. Because it is essential that you should not only read but *follow* the rules that are listed on page 133, at the beginning of the diets.

These rules are common to all WOMAN diets, and an important part of our method. So it's worth while spending a little time discussing the reasons behind them. You will certainly pick up some slimming tips by doing so, and may well dispose of some mistaken notions.

OUR DIETS AND YOUR HEALTH

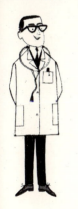

The first rule is one in relation to health. Be sure to consult your doctor before you begin to diet, we advise, unless you are *certain* that you are in perfect health.

This may sound like an excess of caution to anyone who understands even a little elementary nutrition and has read through the diets at the end of the book. Because all that most of them amount to *is* healthy eating.

In fact, from youth to old age, you could quite easily follow one of our average-speed diets which gives a wide choice of food and you would almost certainly be a great deal healthier than the majority of people with their "normal" carbo-hydrate-packed menus.

A genuine improvement in basic health is one of the first things we are constantly noticing about our WOMAN dieters.

We don't stress the health factor to them, because usually they are more concerned at first about changing their appearance. But after a few weeks they almost invariably tell us with some surprise:

"But quite apart from anything else I *feel* so much better—that's the amazing thing. I never realized before that I obviously couldn't have been fully fit for years!"

Often the improvement in health turns out actually to be an even bigger bonus than the improvement in appearance. That was certainly the case with Mrs. M.

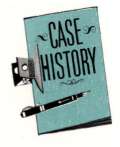

Mrs. M., however kindly you looked at it, was one of those women who had "let herself go". When she came to see us it was obvious that she had given little thought to her appearance. Her dress hem hung down at the back, and her hair was a mess—straight and limp—without even the benefit of a good cut, or a home perm. It quite obviously hadn't had any kind of attention for a considerable length of time.

She brought two little boys with her, and explained that they were the youngest of five. The other three were at school.

Mrs. M. weighed nearly 15 stone, and her attitude to dieting seemed to be backed more by desperation than enthusiasm. Her sister, we gathered, had rather nagged her into coming along to see us. On her own she probably would never have made it.

We knew that it was going to take a great deal of encouragement to get Mrs. M. to keep to her diet. So we asked the sensible sister along to enlist her aid in the campaign.

She told us that life just seemed to have got Mrs. M. down. She had a tremendous amount of work to do for all those children, and didn't have the energy to cope with it. She seemed to drag through the day in a permanent state of exhaustion. And that obviously accounted for the sad state of her appearance and her lack of interest in doing anything about it.

With the help of her sister putting on the pressure on the home front, we managed to get Mrs. M. to keep to her diet in a resigned sort of way. But as the weeks passed, and her weight started to go down, we began to see the first glimmers of enthusiasm.

Actually, Mrs. M. lost weight very well. But it wasn't until the beginning of the third month that we began to notice there was a complete change in her as a person.

By that time our records show that she had lost 1 stone 7 lbs. And this was when she began to smarten up in appearance, and liven up in personality.

"I seem to have more energy," she told us with excitement. "I don't feel as tired and puffed out as I used to be, and I don't get so exhausted by the children."

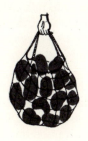

We weren't surprised, we told her. If she had been carrying a shopping bag around all the time containing that 1 stone 7 lbs. worth of weight in potatoes, say, she would certainly have expected to have felt tired. And on her frame it had been "weighing her down" and tiring her out just as surely.

Mrs. M. continued to gain in energy and to become more fit as she lost more weight. When she eventually left us she didn't exactly have a model girl figure, but she weighed 4 stone less than when she had started, and she felt a hundred times better.

The change in appearance had given her a good

psychological boost. But what was still more important, as her sister confirmed, was that now she was fit enough to cope with the demands of an energetic life.

We have heard that the new healthier, livelier Mrs. M. has never looked back!

NOTE OF CAUTION

Now this all helps to explain why we, backed by our medical advisers, have such a great deal of confidence in the health-improving qualities of WOMAN diets. But it doesn't explain the slight note of caution that, you notice, creeps into the first rule.

Well, this is there simply because in the instances of a very few illnesses, a special diet may be necessary from the medical point of view and our own may not be suitable.

Sufferers from some kidney diseases, for instance, may well be required to curtail their intake of proteins. As you know, our diets are generous in proteins.

There's another factor too. We have said that glandular causes for excess weight are relatively rare. But nevertheless they do exist in some cases, and a doctor would be the person to diagnose them.

WOMAN diets are as safe as any diets could be. But it is difficult to believe that there is any such thing as an "excess of caution" when you are dealing with such a vital question as your health. So, if in the slightest doubt at all, you've nothing to lose by being on the safe side with a medical check.

WHY MILK?

We rate the drinking of a daily "half pinta" as one of the most important rules in our diets. Milk is included in every WOMAN diet in this book, and it is there in order to make doubly sure that there can be no element of starvation during the time that you're slimming.

Starvation? Well, of course you couldn't possibly perish on any of the menus we give you. But we want to be certain that your body is not starved of any single one of the nutrients that it needs for good health.

Milk is a good insurance policy for any dieter—because it contains so many important things. It is part protein, part fat and part carbohydrate, and it is particularly rich in a whole range of essential mineral elements—calcium especially.

Of course, that carbohydrate content does mean that milk has to be rationed on your diet. But we have taken it into account as part of our calculations in every case.

So, for the sake of your health, and for the sake of your looks (since they too would suffer if there should be a deficiency of certain nutrients) don't skip milk.

THE DRINKING RULES

We tell you to drink as much as you like of water, unsweetened tea or coffee, meat extract drinks, lemon juice, sugar-free tonic water, and the new sugar-free fruit drinks (but make sure they *are sugar-free*). But we warn you not to drink anything else, (unless it is specifically mentioned in your diet) because those are all the drinks we know of that don't contain some amount of carbohydrate.

As you have learned, it isn't the water in your drinks that can make you fat. It is the other things which have been added.

Alcohol, though not strictly carbohydrate, must be classed as such for the purpose of our diets. It is certainly highly fattening and some alcoholic drinks contain the equivalent of more than half the carbohydrate we would allow on a whole day's menu.

Don't be misled by some of the innocent "slim" sounding names of the other drinks you can buy. "Bitter lemon", for instance sounds safely sugar-free, but in actual fact it does contain sweetening. Even tomato juice and fresh fruit juices contain some carbohydrate.

In the next chapter we will be telling you how to deal with those social occasions when it's "hard to say no" to a drink.

But in connection with your diet it is very important first to get a clear division in your mind between the drinks that will affect your weight, and the drinks that won't.

SUGAR SUBSTITUTES

Unless your diet menu specifically allows a certain amount of sugar (which will then be included in calculations) we have had to ban sugar altogether as a sweetener for all your drinks and cooked dishes.

Instead, we give a specific list of sugar substitutes which can be used freely.

These sugar substitutes are all based on either saccharine or cyclamate. Although the cyclamate-based sweeteners such as Minnim Cubes, Fullsweet, Sweetona, Sucron Mini-Lumps do have a general advantage in pleasantness of taste we would point out that at the time of writing it is felt in some quarters that the safety of taking cyclamates in relatively large amounts has not yet been fully proved. There is no specific evidence to suggest that this is true or that they could contribute to any form of ill-health and nutritionists regard the risk of taking large quantities of sugar as being no less harmful.

We must leave you to make up your own mind

about this subject. We would point out, though, that many people are already eating a certain amount of cyclamate in proprietary sweet foods (not specifically intended for the slimmer) in which it is used as an inexpensive form of sweetening.

We have itemized the saccharine and cyclamate sweeteners, because there are other sugar substitutes which are, in fact, almost as fattening.

We are thinking specifically of sorbitol-based sweeteners. These are often used as sugar-substitutes in diabetic foods. For the purposes of the diabetic, sorbitol acts in a different way from sugar. For the purposes of the normal healthy slimmer, however, it acts in just the same way as sugar and is therefore no help.

In addition to the diabetic foods there are some other proprietary products that boast of their low sugar content and their great value to slimmers, but if you examine the contents label carefully, you will often find that sugar is just replaced by sorbitol.

So, be on the safe side and stick to the sugar substitutes that we recommend.

THE SIZE OF THE PORTION

After you have read the full explanation of our slimming method, you will understand why we can say in the rules:

"Eat as large a portion as you like of any of the foods on the menu, unless an exact portion is specifically stated."

You know, after reading in Chapter 5 about the groups of foods and what each one is like, that it is only those carbohydrate culprits that we are out to beat. And that you are able to eat quite generously from the other groups of foods and still lose the weight you want to.

So you can rest assured that any food that contains an amount of carbohydrate will have been carefully rationed on the menus we give you. The portion will be stated.

Working on that basis, we can safely leave the amount of proteins and fats to you.

In our diets, therefore, we sometimes say "eggs" instead of stating exactly how many—one, or two, it doesn't really matter! And just as long as those carbohydrates are being carefully watched and curtailed it doesn't really matter, either, how much meat and fish and cheese you eat. The same goes, of course, for the many carbohydrate-free vegetables.

Well, we will admit that if you ate these carbohydrate-free foods in really gigantic amounts they could interfere with the success of your dieting campaign.

But people usually just aren't used to eating proteins and fats in such large amounts, and so in almost all cases it is quite safe to follow the demands of your own appetite in deciding on the size of portions of carbohydrate-free foods we mention on our menus.

FACTS ABOUT "SLIMMING BREADS"

Slimming breads and crispbreads come into two basic categories, those which are reduced in carbohydrate and those which are reduced in calories. As the purpose of all the diets in this book is to reduce your daily intake of carbohydrate, only the low-carbohydrate (starch-reduced) breads, crispbreads and rolls must be used. The other varieties could interfere with the careful calculations which ensure your weight loss.

However the low-calorie varieties of breads and crispbreads can be a useful aid to controlling your weight once you have completed your dieting.

You will find the low-carbohydrate breads, loaves, crispbreads and rolls, which are suitable for use with WOMAN diets, listed in Rule 8 on Page 133.

THE MISSED MEALS

The last rule we give you is: "Don't miss out meals". And this is the one that you will probably be the most tempted to break.

Many women tend to regard slimming as a sheer endurance test. The longer they can go hungry, they reason, the quicker they will achieve results, but in practice, this just doesn't work out. In planning our diets we do everything we can to prevent hunger. None of us are tough enough to endure real hunger long, and it's the hungry dieter who gives up or breaks the rules.

Think what happens when you miss out a meal from one of our menus. The chances are that you won't be able to last out until the next meal, and then may well be tempted to eat some snack which will very probably contain more carbohydrate than the missed meal. If you do manage to "last out" the next meal won't satisfy you, and you will eat more than you would otherwise have done.

No, these "starvation tactics" just don't work. You have already read in Chapter 4 the case history of Mrs. P., who tried them and failed.

However, it is more than likely that you will be tempted to miss a meal not through excess enthusiasm, but because you "can't face breakfast".

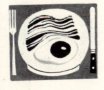

Breakfast, regrettably, has become unfashionable. Pacey people insist on being fragile in the morning on principle. The rest of us are often too concerned with catching the 8.10 or heaving children out of bed, to give it much thought.

Our overweight readers always tell us with a great deal of pride that they never eat breakfast.

It's a pity. Because, as we have to explain so often, good old British bacon-and-eggs and such-like, first thing in the morning, are an almost essential part of successful slimming and in fact we'll go so far as to say that by missing a satisfying breakfast you are probably *gaining* weight. That is not nearly so illogical as it sounds when you consider just how often the abandoned breakfast is compensated for by the mid-morning bun or biscuits, or the couple of slices of toast.

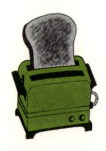

The normal cooked breakfast usually consists of those kindly protein foods. But the toast or the mid-morning snacks are very often packed full of ruinous carbohydrates.

On your diet, a good breakfast will play a tremendous part in controlling your hunger for the rest of the day. Without the breakfast you will find it extremely difficult to stick to the rest of your menu.

We might add that slimmers who insist: "Oh but I couldn't possibly eat breakfast" usually find that they can when once they give it a little try. It doesn't take very long to get into the habit. And when they do, they agree with us that it has made all the difference to the ease of their slimming.

The next thing we are going to consider is what it's like to live with a diet, and the best way of doing this.

Ask yourself these questions if you have tried to diet before and failed:

  1. **When did I stop dieting**—after how many days or weeks?
  2. **Where did I stop dieting**—was it at some special social function?
  3. **Why did I stop dieting**—what was the last straw?

CHAPTER 10
LIVING WITH YOUR DIET

AT THIS STAGE you have probably chosen your WOMAN diet, and been surprised at the generous amount of food it allows.

You may well feel (if you'll pardon such a carbohydrate-filled phrase) that: "It's a piece of cake!"

But wait a minute. Have you bargained for all those slimmer's snares? For snares and temptations there will be, however generous your diet. If you are forewarned they are more easily tackled.

In this chapter you can draw from the experience of thousands of WOMAN slimmers, and learn just when to be on your guard.

SHOULD A SLIMMER TELL?

The biggest snares that you are ever likely to encounter are very often provided by "other people".

Many a diet has gone overboard when a well-meaning but misguided friend or loved-one has protested: "Oh, but I like you just as you are. A bit of extra weight suits you!"

If this kind of comment catches you in a weak moment, you may find yourself agreeing. Subconsciously you may be looking for a good reason to abandon that diet—and here it is! (Next day, you'll be sorry, of course, but by that time you have demolished a box of chocolates and feel that the damage is done. Starting again doesn't seem worth while.)

Should you, then, avoid these pitfalls by being a secret dieter? It isn't difficult on many of the diets in this book which are so closely related to normal eating. We have known many women who managed to "pull it off", and one delightful middle-aged Scottish woman in particular, who managed to keep her dieting a dark secret, even from her own husband. He was amazed to see how her figure was improving, but couldn't for the life of him think why!

However, we would give only a modified "Yes" to this question, because in some cases other people can actually be a help rather than a hindrance.

In these days of increased education about the dangers of excess weight, many people have come to realise that slimming is no joke. And the development and publicizing of really safe diets —in which we feel that WOMAN has played a part—has calmed the fears of many parents about the safety of slimming for their daughters.

A few years ago we would have been surprised to hear a mother suggest to her overweight teen-age daughter: "Joan, you really ought to go on a diet!"

Now we often hear that advice given by enlightened parents.

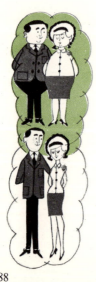

Husbands, too, can be a tremendous help, and we find that they so often are. Let's face it, they have an interest in the matter. Which husband would not prefer a slim and lively, young-looking wife to a large, matronly-looking soul, huffing and puffing around the place?

Many WOMAN dieters have told us that they owe their slimming success almost entirely to the encouragement of their husbands. Often overweight husbands have even agreed to join their wives on a diet. And, incidentally, we should point out at this stage that although we talk about women in this book—because women are our business—there is no reason at all for any of the diets not to be equally successful and safe for men.

"Dieting in pairs" can be a very good plan. If your husband doesn't need to diet, it's not a bad idea to get together with an overweight friend, to gain mutual encouragement and a little healthy competition. But do make sure that you choose someone who is as serious about slimming as you are. A "partner" who swiftly falls by the wayside might well take you with her.

So on the question of diet secrecy we would give this advice: Enlist the support of the people who really care about you. If you are well over a stone overweight, show your family the section of this book which tells about the health dangers of extra weight. If you are a teenager, let your parents read about the safety of WOMAN diets, and in order to give them extra reassurance get your doctor's permission to follow your diet.

But don't talk about your diet to the casual acquaintance, or the "fatty friend" who may secretly prefer to see you stay fatty too.

PARTY
AND PUB
PROBLEMS

In discussing the role of the party or public house in the life of a dieter we must echo the words of the Victorian preacher and sternly warn: "There lies temptation!"

Not that these forms of social activity need necessarily be abandoned during the period of a diet. But they must be handled with some common-sense and firmness.

The two problems they present are these:

1. Almost all drinks served at parties and pubs are fattening.
2. Those "other people" are at their most persuasive in party mood, or after a couple of alcoholic drinks. They may well find pleasure in devoting a whole evening to the demise of your diet.

A little of Stephen Potter's "Lifemanship" will come in useful on these occasions; your essential "ploy" is always to sit with a well-filled glass. As long as you appear to be having a constant supply of drinks the cheerful and well-meaning persuaders will tend to leave you alone. It is unlikely that they will notice how often you actually drink from the glass.

Now we come to the problem of what to put in that glass. Schweppes' Unsweetened Tonic Water, if available, is the drink that immediately suggests itself, because with this you can go on safely sipping all evening without any damage to your diet.

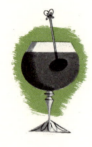

Other drinks commonly available at parties and pubs all contain a certain amount of carbo-hydrate. But for dieting purposes tomato juice is the least lethal. A couple of glasses of this would have a carbohydrate content roughly equivalent to that of a thin slice of bread. If you linger over them all evening, and perhaps cut out two or three crispbreads over the next few days of your diet, no harm will be done.

(To satisfy the person who obviously feels strongly that you can't be enjoying yourself with-out some alcoholic assistance, you could always hint that the tomato juice contains a vodka!)

But how you cope with these occasions depends to some extent on how frequently they occur in your life. The woman who seldom goes to parties or public houses would not be ruining her slim-ming chances by drinking one glass of wine (less fattening than spirits) at the one big social occasion which crops up during her diet.

For the purposes of that big "company dinner" or anniversary outing, it would be a good idea in fact to change just for one day to the "Dieting by Numbers" diet in this book, see page 145, which allows for a small amount of alcohol as long as it is taken into the calculations. This would also give you a wider choice of food from the menu.

However, the woman who often attends social functions where alcohol is served might be wise to curtail them during her diet, unless she is very sure indeed of her own determination and the strength of her will-power.

THE DANGER WEEKS

Now we come to those special periods during a diet when determination is most needed—the "danger weeks". If we could chart on a graph the strength-of-will of almost any dieter, we should see it taking a sharp swoop down on the third week, and probably another dip round about the sixth.

The third week of a diet is the one that really separates the winners from the losers. The reasons are fairly obvious when you remember that the first week often shows a quite sensational weight loss, while the second week rarely produces a loss of more than half that amount.

So the slimmer often starts on the third week of her diet with a certain feeling of disappointment. She begins to think that this diet is going to take an awful long time—and perhaps allows herself to wonder if it's really worth it. At this stage she is very vulnerable to the sort of temptations we have just discussed.

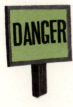

The best antidote to third-week-blues is to be prepared for them. It's usually the unexpected obstacle that trips us up!

And this is where the members of the family who are "on your team" in this slimming campaign can really help you a good deal with their encouragement and enthusiasm.

By the sixth week the girl who had only a stone

91

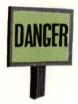

or less to lose will probably have reached, or almost reached, her target. She'll be feeling pretty pleased with herself, so we needn't worry about her. But for the woman with two stone or more to shed this will be just about half-way mark, and another rather tricky period.

A little boredom may set in. Not necessarily boredom with the food, which as you know, can be extremely varied on many WOMAN diets. But simply boredom with the whole idea of dieting.

The thing to tell yourself at this stage is: "Hold on for a while—even if it's only for another couple of weeks!" Because by the end of those two weeks you should start to reap the rewards that will carry you sailing on to achieve your weight loss target.

People will really begin to see that you have lost weight. Your family will not have noticed much difference during the first few weeks because of the gradual process of weight reduction. But suddenly someone you haven't seen for quite a while will stop in surprise and exclaim: "Aren't you looking marvellous—you're so slim! Whatever have you been doing?"

Your clothes will start to feel loose. At last you can have the pleasure of actually "taking in" seams! You start to feel much livelier and fitter. And you'd swear that the stairs have become much less steep than they ever used to be!

At this stage that boredom you felt will be replaced by a real feeling of exhilaration, and you can safely assume that you are over the last hump. You're nearly there!

WHEN YOU'RE TEMPTED

Quite apart from the danger weeks there are those moments of temptation, which can crop up any time, when you have no intention of abandoning

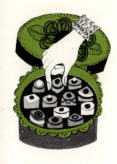

your diet, but feel that you absolutely must have just one teeny-weeny chocolate cream.

Should you succumb to temptation just this once? After all, you might reason, one chocolate cream isn't going to undo a whole week's slimming effort.

You are quite right, of course, but the trouble with one teeny-weeny chocolate cream is it invariably leads to another teeny-weeny chocolate cream—and then another.

It's just like trying to give up smoking. That one cigarette wouldn't matter in itself except that it always leads to more.

What's to be done then? Do you just grit your teeth and try not to feel hungry?

There's an easier answer than that. If you feel hungry or even if you just feel tempted, treat yourself to a tasty nibble that won't spoil your diet.

There are a number of things that can be nibbled freely during a WOMAN diet. For the cheese-lover, cheese is the obvious answer. Keep a good supply of your favourite type in the pantry for moments when you want to spoil yourself without spoiling your figure.

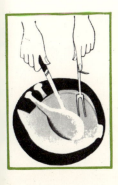

Any type of meat or fish can be used to cope with a hunger pang (a cold chicken in the fridge would be a real slimming investment). Or you could eat a hard-boiled egg, or a stick of celery.

For a complete list of "free-to-nibble" foods you can refer to the "Foods You Can Eat Freely" section of the "Dieting by Numbers" diet, which is on page 147.

What you must avoid, however, is eating other things which you just imagine to be non-fattening in between meals. WOMAN diet experts have often had to play detective to track down this culprit behind the apparent temporary failure of a diet. The puzzle of Margaret X was one case in point.

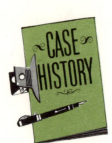

Margaret was a lively girl with the unusual job of being a chauffeur. No one could have been more enthusiastic about losing weight than she was.

She weighed just under 11 stone when she started on her diet, and was determined to get down to the 9½ stone which was more in keeping with her height and build.

When she came to us for a weight check at the end of the first week she had lost just under 2 lbs. Not bad—but not marvellous for the starting week!

The second week showed a loss of only ¾ lb., and when the third week's loss was about the same we began to realise that something was wrong. This was a fairly strict diet that Margaret was following and should have been achieving faster results.

We questioned Margaret closely.

"Honestly," she protested, "I'm keeping right to my diet. I haven't cheated at all!"

We continued to puzzle over Margaret's slow weight loss, until eventually one day she offered to give one of the WOMAN diet staff a lift home in her car.

Our colleague stumbled over a large paper bag as she got into her seat.

"Sorry," said Margaret, "it's my apple bag. I munch them when I'm driving alone. It helps me when I'm feeling peckish."

Then she noticed the expression on our colleague's face.

"But they aren't fattening—*are* they. . . ?"

Because the fallacy that fruit has no fattening

content is such a popular one, Margaret had just taken it for granted and hardly given her apple-eating a thought. She had never associated it in her mind with her slow rate of weight loss.

She was genuinely surprised when we explained that *all* fruit, with the exception of lemons, has some carbohydrate content. Not a large amount of carbohydrate when you consider it in relation to bread, potatoes and most sweet things. But quite enough for the quantity of apples she ate to slow down her weight loss.

IT PAYS TO BE ORGANIZED

From the temptation problems that we have just discussed, you will see one of the reasons good organization is essential to a dieter. If she has thought ahead and set aside that tasty non-fattening nibble she'll sail through the difficult moment without any danger to her dieting. But if all the pantry contains in the way of snacks is a box of biscuits, you can imagine what happens!

Well-planned shopping is a number one priority. Many a diet is abandoned simply because shopping has not been done, and that handy old stand-by—perhaps a tin of baked beans —is the only thing available.

This vital factor was taken into account in our questions which lead you to your ideal diet. The woman who is inclined to get a little disorganized in her shopping will find that the diet with a repeating one-week menu makes things easier. She can order the same food each week, and will soon find she is getting into an easy routine.

HOW TO CHECK YOUR WEIGHT

Now here's the question that every dieter asks: "How often should I get weighed?"

If she owns a pair of bathroom scales she probably asks the question, but takes little notice of

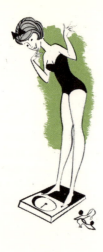

the answer. She just can't resist getting on those scales every day, probably several times a day.

This is where she is making a big mistake—and we hope that we can talk her out of it. Because this can be not only discouraging but downright misleading.

One of the reasons is that during the course of a day our weight does not stay constant. It travels up and down to a surprising degree. Try a one-day test yourself and you will see how much it really does vary.

Late in the evening you might weigh more than you did in the morning; after a meal your weight may temporarily rise by nearly a pound. During an interval of just a few minutes you may find that you have dropped half a pound in weight simply because you have emptied your bowel or bladder.

Because of these hour-to-hour changes the small amount of weight that you may lose in just one day cannot be accurately recorded. But a weekly weight loss is going to be big enough to overshadow these factors, and give you at least a clear indication of how you are getting on.

So get weighed once-a-week only. And try to get weighed at the same time of day.

If you own bathroom scales, first thing in the morning, before you dress, is the ideal time. If you don't, try to make your visits to the chemist's scales at the same time of day, and wear the same clothes each time you go.

You may suspect that the shop scales you use are not correctly adjusted. But this doesn't really matter as long as you use the *same* scales each week. The important thing is not to record your correct weight, but your weight *loss*—and this they should still do, even if they may actually be adding or taking off a pound or so all the time.

However, you will remember learning in a previous chapter that at certain times—and especially just before the monthly period—all weighing scales can "tell lies". Therefore, throughout your diet it is a good idea to make weekly double checks with tape-measure as well as scales.

Before you start, take measurements and note them down. Measure around your bust, around your abdomen, your waist, your upper and lower hips, thighs and ankles. Check these measurements and note them down again each week of your diet—preferably doing your measurement check on the same day every time, say Monday, to give an encouraging start to a new week.

Then, if you come to the time when you could swear you had lost weight, but those scales just won't move, you can reassure yourself with the tape-measure.

A FREQUENT PROBLEM

As a footnote to this chapter we will deal with one little problem that is quite often mentioned by our dieters. And this is a certain tendency towards constipation in the early weeks of a diet.

When this occurs we remind the dieter that she is probably not taking in the same bulk of food that her body has become used to, and therefore there is not the same amount of waste matter to excrete. There is no need to start worrying if she does not have a daily bowel movement.

The change of eating habits has probably contributed to this problem, which generally solves itself in a few weeks when the body has become fully adjusted to this change. However, where it causes any worry or discomfort we recommend Senocott.

We know of no other health problems that

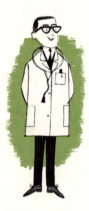

could be caused by our dieting. Even the minor ones, like tiredness and lack of energy, which women who are used to crash diets have come to expect, are eradicated by the generous allowance of varied foods we provide on our menus.

So if you do feel unwell during your slimming campaign, don't fall into the trap of thinking: "It must just be the diet!" Check with your doctor to find the true cause.

CHAPTER 11

CLOTHES THAT HELP YOU "CHEAT"

SO FAR, we have not yet touched on the subject of "spot reduction".

We do realize, however, that very many women are most anxious to lose weight mainly from one particular part of the body—perhaps the hips, seat, or bust.

Just how much can our slimming methods help with this problem?

Well, first we must consider *why* your figure is out of proportion, and has the extra, unwanted bulk in certain areas.

This is often partly a problem of fat, for quite frequently bodies have a tendency to store fat in particular regions—notably the hips and breasts where women are concerned, and the abdomen in men.

But this need not be the whole cause, nor even the only cause.

It is a fact that many a woman, who is otherwise as slim as she would like to be, can never achieve a perfectly balanced figure simply because of wide hip-bones, and there is nothing at all that any diet can do about it.

Unusual development of particular muscle groups can be another factor. This is often the reason that an otherwise slim girl may have disproportionately large thighs.

We can't blame bones or muscles for a large bust, but in addition to any excess weight, some heredity factor may be partly responsible for making the breasts large in proportion to the rest of a woman's body.

In discussing what part our diets can play in improving the proportions of your figure we must consider the women with these problems in two separate groups.

Women who have an all-over weight

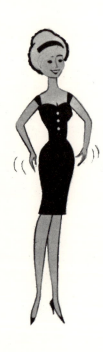

problem, but are especially bulky in one particular area, belong to the first and largest group, which would actually include the majority of over-weight women. Very few manage to retain perfectly-balanced proportions.

It is here that our diets can—and do—play an enormous part in improving figure-balance. For the woman who is generally overweight can most often attribute her particularly large hips, seat or bust mainly to the excess fat storage there is in that area.

As she starts to slim, her proportions may not immediately show any improvement. The fat will be disappearing gradually from all parts of the body. But after a certain length of time the body will have to draw on the extra supplies in that particular problem area.

We find the vast majority of our slimmers have improved their proportions by the time they have completed their diet campaigns. But this does not necessarily mean that they have become perfectly proportioned. Bone structure, muscles and here-dity may well have played a small part, too, in determining what their shape shall be. And these are things that are not going to change.

The second group, that we shall be discussing, consists of those slim girls with the one-area figure problem—like those girls we mentioned who have slim bodies but disproportionately large thighs.

In this group, bone and muscle are most likely to be the culprits.

You can check this for yourself by feeling the bulky area.

If it feels soft, and gives to the touch, a fat deposit might well be the problem, and a diet could provide the solution. But if it feels firm and hard, it would suggest that bones and muscles are the cause of your one-area problem and that a slimming diet is not going to be a great deal of help to you.

Well, that would certainly seem to be that, for a number of people who have always longed for perfect proportions. We can't suggest a method of slimming muscles and bones!

But we do know the way to help you keep your proportion problems a secret known only to you, and present the appearance of a well-balanced figure to the outside world.

"Cheat" those extra inches away by careful choice of the clothes you wear. It's very easy when you know the basic principles that lie behind this way of dressing.

In this chapter we are going to supply the fashion know-how for correcting proportion problems. And at the end of the chapter—for the benefit of those of you who want to reap the maximum number of compliments for those new, slim figures—we will tell you about the clothes that will help to make you look even slimmer than you have become.

TIPS FOR THE TOP-HEAVY

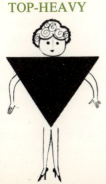

If a large bust happens to be your special figure problem, and hips and seat are fairly trim, avoid high necklines, elaborate collars and tight belts, and wear any bright-coloured clothes below the waist only.

Skirts can be gathered, pleated or flared. If you want to choose a straight style, go for a bold pattern, or a bulky or textured fabric that attracts the eye.

Coats and suits are best if they widen out towards the hem: coats should be full-length because the three-quarter kind demand a slim skirt, and a silhouette (wrong for you) that tapers in to the knees; suit jackets are best if between waist and hip-bone length. Choose your sleeves raglan or softly shaped, and keep any eye-catching details that you want well below waist level. Low-slung patch pockets and gaily braided hems are just the job!

Dresses should follow the rules for skirts and the bodices should be kept plain. Low-set neck-lines and sleeveless styles help to cut width—particularly if necklines and armholes are edged with darker bands of colour. Shift shapes, simple and sleeveless, are always the most flattering for the younger woman.

Blouses can be tucked in to let your skirts or trousers look more important, but sweaters that cling and emphasize your shape are by no means to be recommended!

Accessories are best kept unobtrusive if they're to be worn above the waist. Brooches displayed on the bosom, or large dangly strings of beads are definitely not for you.

TIPS FOR THE BROAD-BASED

If you're larger below the waist than above it (the good old familiar British "pear shape" so many of us are heirs to), then avoid gathered, ruched or pleated skirts, short jackets, raglan sleeves, double breasting and large cuffs. Keep the brighter colours of your wardrobe to garments you wear above the waist, such as blouses, jacket and sweaters.

Skirts should be kept simple and straight as much as possible, slightly eased or flared. For extra ease of movement, if necessary, you could have inverted pleats at the back and front, but never consider having them the whole way round. Dark insets down the side of light-coloured skirts, or a front inset on a dark one, will act as hip trimmers.

Coats and jackets can be straight at the back and shaped at the front, three-quarter length or long, but you should never choose a belted version; Princess lines that have high pockets and wide necklines are very much more flattering to your type of figure.

Dresses flatter you most when they have a smooth outline. When the bust is very small, in proportion to the hips, both tunics worn over sweaters and under-bust gathering can add needed bulk above the waist.

Accessories can be bright and bold: large hats, scarves, brooches and chunky necklaces; but keep shoes, stockings and handbags simple.

Separates should have important, eye-catching tops, straight jerkins. Don't tuck your sweaters and blouses into skirts or trews as this would only emphasise the hips.

SPECIAL-AREA PROBLEMS

Too large bust or hips are far and away the most common of the proportion problems. But some women carry their figure-spoiling bulk on certain other areas of the body.

A large seat often combines with large hips; the same clothes-cunning can "correct" both.

Some women, however, have fairly narrow hips and a large, "low-slung" seat—what our fashion girls would call a "sway back". Here, the best solution would be tops worn outside skirts and slacks, low-waisted dresses, and blouses and jackets which are just slightly bloused at the back —always be careful not to wear clinging blouses and sweaters or tight belts.

Thick thighs can easily be disguised by skirts with a slight flare. They are more of a problem in slacks, and here a three-quarter-length jacket is the best solution. When you're buying swimming gear, choose a swimsuit that has a little skirt.

A short waist is another thing that can at times spoil the proportioning of the body, and in this case the answer is always to wear long, straight jackets, sweaters and blouses—and Empire-line dresses if you are "pear-shaped" as well. Avoid belts on the waist.

SLIMMING CLOTHES

Now we come to the points on clothes that have an all-over slimming value.

We like to think that these are going to be kept in mind by the fairly slim in order to make them look *very* slim. We hope, that after reading this book, no woman is ever going to be content to remain fat!

Fabrics, patterns and colours play the biggest part in achieving our object.

Here is your guide:

Choose these minimizers: small prints and small checked ginghams, flecked or mottled designs and muted colours (warm plum, for instance, rather than pillar box red).

Go for the smooth, matt-surfaced materials that are closely woven and may have vertical interest in the weave as well. In this class are linen, flannel, double jersey, gaberdine, the fine tweeds and worsteds; tussore and shantung, which are coarser and less shiny than other silks; and any of the synthetics which resemble what we have suggested. The least fattening furs are the smooth ones, like antelope, seal, otter and pony skin. Suede is ideal too.

Avoid these inch-adders: splashy, all-over floral designs, large check patterns and bright colours. These are the materials that also have a tendency to make you look larger than life: bulky, heavy tweeds, mohairs, corduroys, velvets and lacy wools, shiny satins, chiffons, taffetas, glazed cottons, polished brocades, thick and long-haired furs.

SIMPLE STYLES Simplicity is going to be your greatest ally in making you look really sleek—and, which is certainly a matter to be considered, in showing off a newly slimmed figure! Frills, ruffles and unnecessary beading, buttons and bows will only add bulk.

A little understatement can say a surprising amount for you. A trim little self-coloured dress in one of the minimizing materials we mention above needs no additions to tell its own most flattering story.

When you have eventually become really slim, the dress can be perfectly figure-hugging if you want it to be.

But before that, it's much wiser to make certain that it is "figure-skimming" only, straight, or with just a semi-fitted waist.

Clothes that make you look taller also make you look slimmer. So unless an extra inch or two at head level is one of your problems, and you tend to feel at times that you're something of a giraffe, go for the long look.

Pay particular attention to hemlines, for skirts even an inch too long will make *you* seem a whole inch shorter.

Go for a toning, rather than contrasting, colour scheme from top to toe. Separates are as good for your purpose as all-one-piece dresses and coats *only* when they are kept to the same colour tone. Follow this principle even with your accessories. Hats should be the same colour as your outfit, and stockings and shoes should be neutral for an all-of-a-piece look.

Any downward stripe tends to be lengthening and slimming. So a fasten-down-the middle dress, with buttons or a braided edge, would be a particularly good buy for you.

Make sure that you see yourself from all angles in the dress-shop mirror before you buy anything. Take a frank friend along, if you can. And—most important of all—never try to "squeeze a quart into a pint pot". That's the best way we know to look fat.

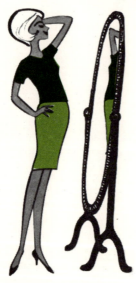

CHAPTER 12
THE SHAPING AIDS

BECAUSE OUR DIETS are based on normal everyday foods we hope that they will cost you only a little effort—and very little extra money. But, be warned—what they *will* cost you is the price of a new set of foundation garments.

After you've managed to lose all that weight it would be a crying shame not to make the most of your wonderful new figure. And it will be only good, well-fitting foundation garments that show off the slimmer curves you're so pleased with to their very best advantage.

When overweight readers are slimming under our supervision, we always get tremendous pleasure from watching them gradually becoming more attractive as each week goes by.

But the big day for us, and for them, is the day right at the end of their slimming campaigns when they call in to see us, wearing their new figure-fitting foundation garments under their smart new outfits.

That's when we find ourselves rushing round the office telling our colleagues: "Look, you really must come and see Mrs. T. You just won't believe that she's the same woman we saw only three months ago!"

A good figure depends on four factors— weight, proportion, firmness and shape. Foundation garments can take care of the shaping for you, and this will make all the difference to the new look of your figure.

During a diet, unless money is no object, most of us just have to put up with the old foundation garments from fatter days. Since a perfect fit is essential, it would be silly to buy new ones while the figure is changing—and of course the old ones will gradually become looser and less effective as the pounds are shed, week by week. That is one of the reasons we always see such a sensational change in our dieters after an end-of-campaign session with a corsetière.

These garments make such a difference that we would certainly give you this advice: If you can't afford to buy new clothes and new foundations right away, then take in your old *clothes* to fit your new figure, and spend what money you can afford on buying a new bra and girdle, or else an all-in-one corselette.

Don't try "taking in" foundation garments. Only a trained expert can do this efficiently. To give you the proper support they must have correct balance—and any tucks that you made would interfere with this.

HOW TO CHOOSE

The soundest bit of advice that we can give you about choosing these new foundation garments is this: Get help. There is plenty of expert help readily available. Most of the department stores have experienced corsetières in their lingerie departments—and they are there to help you to find a perfect fit.

Some people feel shy of allowing a stranger into their changing cubicle. And you may well have acquired this aversion when you were fat and self-conscious about your figure. However, try to remember that the corsetière is used to seeing undressed people of all shapes and sizes—probably shapes and sizes that would make your worst ones look good and your figure now is quite different from what it was before you started your slim-campaign.

Like the doctor, she is a disinterested person, concerned only with doing her job. And we find that most corsetières have the tact to say: "Try this one on, and just ring the bell when you are ready," when they see any signs of shyness in one of their customers.

It is possible, through firms like Spirella who give a personal service, to have a corsetry fitting in your own home. There is probably a trained representative in your area who would come round to take your measurements, and supply you with made-to-measure garments.

Buying without trying is all very well for a girl who stays the same size and has discoverd the bra and girdle that are ideal for her. There are some chain stores which haven't any changing facilities but do an extremely good line in foundation garments of all kinds bought straight over the counter.

But, after the shape of your figure has radically changed through slimming, a lengthy trying-on session is essential—to achieve perfection. Even knowing what your exact measurements are is not sufficient, because the shapes of people, and the shapes of the garments which suit them, differ just as much as the sizes.

BUYING A BRA

Before buying a bra it is a good idea to get an idea of your basic measurements, so that you know what sizes to start trying on. To do this, run a tape-measure around your rib-cage just under the bust (under your clothes, of course). Now add 5 inches to those measurements. This will indicate the basic size of bra you need—32 in., 34 in., 36 in. and so on.

Next measure around the fullest part of the bust. The difference between the two measurements indicates your cup fitting: a 5 inch difference usually means an A cup, 6 inches a B cup, 7 inches a C cup, and 8 inches a D cup.

Armed with this information, go to the shop or

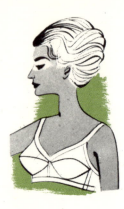

store which offers the widest possible range of foundation garments, and ask a corsetière to help you select some different makes and styles for you to try on.

If your bust is still on the generous side, look out for special supporting features in whichever bra you select.

These can consist of wire frames which rim the lower half of the bra cups; boning at the sides; stiffening material in the under half of the cups; or a cross-stitched double thickness of material in the under half of the cup.

A deep bra is often a good idea for the larger bust. It might be bordered with a firm elasticated section, or with a wide band of material. Or it could extend right to the waist with light boning for extra control.

Wide shoulder straps are another golden rule for extra comfort—particularly the stretchy kind which are now widely available, and are so good for wearing with wide-necked dresses because you can push the straps over and they stay in position.

Take about half a dozen bras into the fitting room. And if you don't immediately find one that is perfect in every way, send for more. Don't be tempted to buy in a rush.

To try on a bra, lean forward so that your breasts fall naturally into the cups. Then straighten up to fasten the back before you start to adjust shoulder straps.

The straps should not have to be tight to give the necessary uplift. If you find that they are, the basic construction is wrong for you, and you must turn to another.

You will see exactly what we mean about widely differing shapes when you start to try a bra on. Sometimes the cups will be too pointed for the shape of your breasts and you will see loose material at the centre of the cup. This would cause a bad outline under clothes.

Others may seem to fit the breast shape fairly well, but you will find that they create a roll of fat under the arm. Reject these too.

Another thing to look for is good division. Make sure that the bra is constructed to hold the breasts gently but firmly apart, and that the material between the cups fits well and doesn't jut out away from you.

When something is wrong with those you try on, the experienced corsetière will know where to lay hands on another bra that will solve the problem. It's well worth spending a little time on finding the perfect shape and size.

BUYING A GIRDLE OR CORSET

When you buy girdles or corsets, do remember that nowadays foundations need not have a cast-iron look to give firm control. Multi-boned corsets made of mainly rigid material are still available, but only to satisfy the insistence of women who have grown accustomed to them, and just can't believe that anything with a lighter look could give the control they want.

We are against these inflexible garments on two counts. Firstly they tend to give an ageing "packaged" look to the wearer—far from the young lithe look that you can now aim for with your slimmer figure.

And, secondly, they encourage muscle slackness. Women who wear them continually tend to rely on them too much. They let their own muscles go completely slack inside this "armour plating" and by the time they reach middle age their bodies have become loose and flabby.

If you have been wearing a corset like this, now

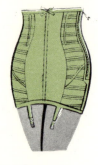

is the time, after your slimming and exercising campaign, for you to make the change to a modern corset or a firm girdle.

Modern corsets have only a minimum of boning, and are made mainly of light flexible materials like Lycra and Vyrene, which move with the muscles. The rigid material is usually confined to a centre panel down the front.

You have to rely on your own muscle control a little more with these garments. And that is a very good thing, because it will help you to keep your muscles firm, and your body young-looking.

If you choose a girdle rather than a corset, look for the light but helpful reinforcements. The best modern girdles tend to rely on a double thickness of light stretchy material across back and front (often in a criss-cross style) to give this extra control, rather than panels of rigid material.

Any fitter worth her salt will insist on measuring you herself for these garments. Most of them insist that we can't do it properly ourselves.

When trying on a corset, remember that the short-waisted corset should start just a little below the waist, because it will rise when you sit down. The high-waisted one, which usually has light-boning at the top, should fit so that it lies lower at the back that at the front.

Both types should curve in snugly below the seat to give a good fit and prevent them rising.

Remember that these days corsets are made in masses of different sizes to suit every figure in every way. At one time many women would put up with, say, a loose waist, to get a garment which gave a good fit around hips or seat. But this is no longer necessary. Make sure that the corset fits snugly but comfortably all over.

To make sure a girdle or corset is comfortable,

check on it sitting as well as standing. Look in the mirror to see that it gives you a nice flat tummy and a neat seat. And check also to see that it doesn't push out rolls of flesh at the thighs or waist. (Long-legged pantie girdles, incidentally, are the best garments to choose if you have to cope with a thick-thigh problem.)

There is no point at all in trying to squeeze into a size too small. This will only make you bulge out in other places, and make your figure look worse instead of better.

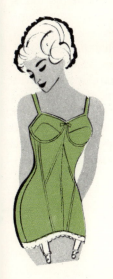

BUYING ALL-IN-ONES

All-in-one foundation garments which extend from the bust to the thighs, are usually referred to as corselettes. They can do a splendid re-shaping job for the newly slimmed figure.

But, again, it is important to ensure that they are light-looking garments with large areas of fine stretchy material and a minimum of boning. The more rigid garments will always tend to give a very solid appearance to any figure.

These days corselettes need not necessarily be made-to-measure because a large corsetry department can stock them in a huge variety of sizes. However, the help of an expert fitter is absolutely imperative. The garment may need some adjustment to give you a perfect fit, but the large stores are able to do these alterations in an expert way.

Of course, a made-to-measure service, supplied by firms like Spirella, would be equally good.

To try on a corselette, first cross your legs and clench your buttocks. The corselette should be doubled-over, held with finger-tips (careful, if your nails are long!), and then drawn over the hips with one quick movement. When the lower half is in position, draw up the top. Fastenings should be worked upwards, and zips should avoid hip bones. When fastening your stockings, follow the slant of the suspenders and fasten the back ones first.

Look for a perfect fit by checking the same points that you would with a separate bra and girdle. See that the cups fit correctly at the centre, with no loose material, that there is good division, and no rolls of flesh pushed up under the arms or down at the thighs. And make sure that you are comfortable sitting as well as standing.

CARING FOR FOUNDATION GARMENTS

You will probably get better value in the long run from your foundation garments if you can manage to buy more than one of each. This makes really regular laundering more sure and simple. Oddly enough, frequent laundering *helps* to preserve the life of these garments, because it is perspiration which tends to rot the elasticated materials.

Many manufacturers are now advertising bras and girdles which come to no harm in the washing machine, and these are a particularly good buy for people who find hand-washing an extra chore.

We think that it is worth spending as much as you can afford on really top-class foundation garments. An inexpensive dress can look marvellous when you are wearing the right things underneath.

CHAPTER 13
TONE UP AS YOU SLIM DOWN

WE HAVE ALREADY EXPLAINED the part exercises are to play in your campaign for a new figure: they will be more concerned with firming muscles than actually shedding fat. But don't underestimate their value to your looks—particularly if you are past the teens and twenties stage.

Just consider what factors tend to make a woman look older than she wants to look. Excess weight is one thing. Not just because it is associated so often with a matronly person, but because it also leads to old-looking, effort-filled movement. More about that later.

The second thing you may think of is wrinkles. Well, they come to us all eventually—although, of course, a routine of regular beauty care, geared to your type of skin, does help to keep them at bay as long as possible.

But if you are really observant you will have noted that loose, flabby muscles are probably the biggest culprit of them all.

Think of those give-away areas that tell so many tales about age. Old-looking arms, for instance, with soft loose muscles at the top back. And then there's the soft tummy, and the general all-over sag of the body.

You've probably been amazed by the still girlish figures of some of those no-longer young stars of stage and screen (think of Marlene Dietrich!). In your fireside frankness by the TV screen, you may remark that their faces may look a little older, but their figures look exactly the same as they did twenty (or thirty) years ago.

We are sure that these remarkable women owe their young figures to more than just dieting. They must exercise to keep so lithe and firm.

Of course, we are not advocating exercises for only the over-thirties. Teens and twenties who have been overweight need them just as much to get back a really pussycat sleekness.

In this chapter we illustrate exercises which we suggest you should make part of a daily routine while you are dieting. But first, a word about ordinary, everyday movements. While you have been overweight you have probably acquired bad habits in movement and deportment.

If you are carrying round a couple of extra stone it's hard not to look as if you are! You tend to drag yourself upstairs by the banister, walk with a slight stoop, sit down with a flop.

When you have lost this extra weight on your WOMAN diet, this problem may correct itself. You will feel livelier and lighter and your movements may be livelier and lighter. But some of the old ways may linger on out of sheer habit.

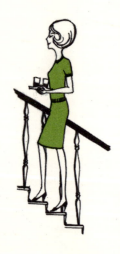

So take stock of your movements and your general deportment. Remind yourself that *now you are lighter*. You can walk up stairs, your back erect, without even touching the rail. You can bend your knees and lower yourself lightly into a chair. You can walk with your shoulders comfortably straight (no need to hold them ram-rod stiff to keep them back), and with your head upright, instead of poking forward.

Start learning good habits now, and you'll have become more attractive in yet another way by the time you've reshaped your figure.

The exercises which, together, add up to an all-over figure-trimming routine begin on the facing page. Repeat each one as advised. But if you are over forty, unused to exercise, or very heavily overweight, it would be wise to work them up only very gradually. Start by spending only four or five minutes daily on your exercise routine, then add an extra minute each day.

EXERCISES

FOR LEGS AND FEET

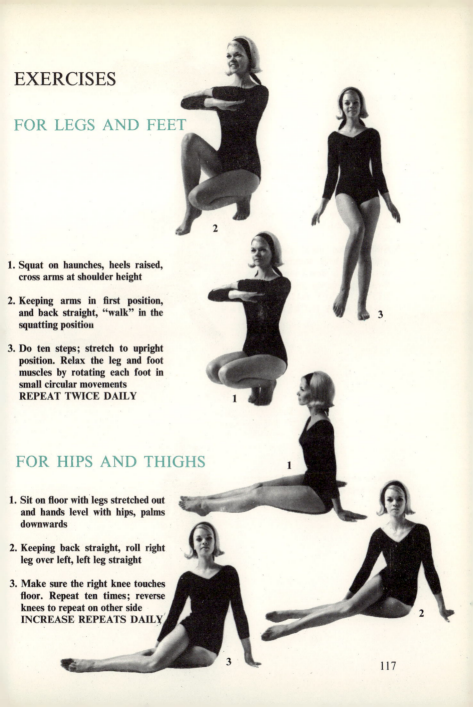

2

3

1

1. Squat on haunches, heels raised, cross arms at shoulder height

2. Keeping arms in first position, and back straight, "walk" in the squatting position

3. Do ten steps; stretch to upright position. Relax the leg and foot muscles by rotating each foot in small circular movements
   REPEAT TWICE DAILY

1

FOR HIPS AND THIGHS

1. Sit on floor with legs stretched out and hands level with hips, palms downwards

2. Keeping back straight, roll right leg over left, left leg straight

3. Make sure the right knee touches floor. Repeat ten times; reverse knees to repeat on other side
   INCREASE REPEATS DAILY

2

3

TO FIRM BUSTLINE

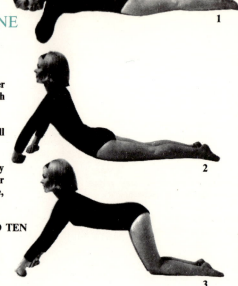

1. Lie flat on tummy, hands under shoulders, palms on floor with fingers pointing inwards

2. Push body up from the waist till arms are straight

3. Still pushing back, raise body with knees bent. Return to floor position to a slow count of five, breathing in as you go down **REPEAT ONCE DAILY, GRADUALLY INCREASE TO TEN**

TO TRIM WAISTLINE

1. Stand straight, with legs apart, hands held loosely at sides

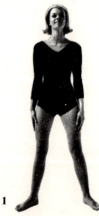

2. Raise left arm slowly, letting ▶ hand slide down right leg

TO TRIM MIDRIFF

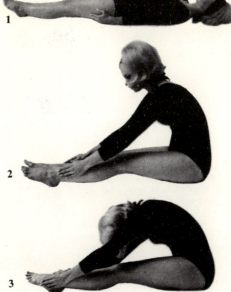

1. Lie flat on your back with arms straight at sides, feet together

2. Take a deep breath, then sit up slowly and lean forward, pushing arms down sides of legs

3. Try to touch knees with your head, keeping legs straight. Uncurl slowly, return to first position, breathing out as you do so
INCREASE GRADUALLY TO FIVE REPEATS

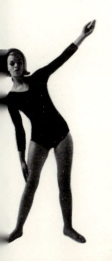

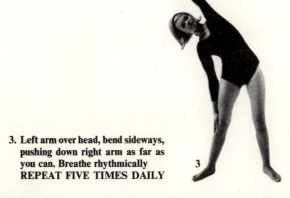

3. Left arm over head, bend sideways, pushing down right arm as far as you can. Breathe rhythmically
REPEAT FIVE TIMES DAILY

119

TO FIRM
UPPER ARMS

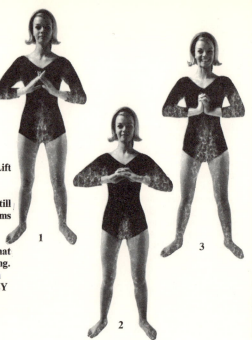

1

3

1. **Stand straight, legs apart. Lift elbows, lock fingers together**

2. **Hands at midriff-level, fingers still locked firmly, jerk your palms outwards**

3. **Push hands together hard so that you feel arm muscles tightening. Return hands to second position REPEAT TEN TIMES DAILY**

2

TO BRACE TUMMY MUSCLES

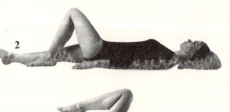

1

1. **Lie on your back, legs straight, palms downwards on floor**

2. **Bend left leg at knee, keeping other leg quite straight**

2

3. **Bring knee to chest. Lower leg and repeat with right leg. Breathe rhythmically during exercise REPEAT TEN TIMES DAILY**

3

CHAPTER 14

STAY AS SLIM AS YOU ARE

WE HOPE that by the time you have reached this late stage in the book you have resolved to lose weight, have flipped ahead to find your own personal WOMAN diet, and can hardly wait to do battle with the carbohydrates.

But if we were to suggest that you might spend a little time considering how to keep slim after you get slim . . . well, you might very well say: "Look, let me lose the weight first, and then I'll worry about that!"

Fair enough. We suggest that you read, or at least re-read, this chapter *after* you have achieved your weight loss target.

For at that stage you will be so delighted with your new slim figure that any hints we can give you on how to "stay as slim as you are" will have rated a new importance.

So we'll assume that now you are slim—as slim as you ever wanted to be. Your diet has achieved its object, and now you can forget about it, if you want to.

But what are your chances of staying as slim as this in the future?

Well they are very good indeed if you use a little common sense and give a little thought to it. From time to time we have taken a survey on former WOMAN dieters and discovered, to our great satisfaction, that many of them have managed to stay slim. Although a few, of course, have fallen by the wayside.

Let's make sure that you are not one of those who join the few by the wayside.

SHOPPING IS IMPORTANT

As we explained in an earlier chapter, it's at this point that your better-behaved appestat is now going to take over and help to control your weight, because by slimming on a WOMAN diet you have re-trained it into better eating habits, and you should no longer have such a desire for those fattening foods as you had before.

However, your appestat does need a little amount of co-operation from you. If it suggests that a meat and vegetable dish would be nice for lunch, but all you've got on the shelves of your pantry happens to be tins of baked beans, bread and sweet biscuits—well, you just aren't giving it a chance to keep you in line!

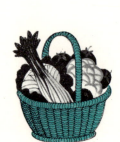

We emphasized the importance of organized shopping in getting slim, and now we are going to emphasize it again as part of keeping slim.

It's a funny thing about housewives . . . they spend a large part of their time planning meals for their families, but rarely give a thought to planning meals for themselves.

Hands up those who—before their diets—just ate "anything that was going" or "something that needed eating up" for lunch!

We rarely come across any housewives who give the slightest thought to planning the meals they eat when they are by themselves, while the rest of the family are out at work or school.

And so now, whether you are a housewife or a single girl, we want you to start giving some careful thought in advance to your meals.

Choose the things that you like most out of the mainly protein and vegetable foods that you have become used to eating, and remember to shop for them specifically. This will play a tremendous part in keeping you slim.

To help you in this we have compiled you a special weight-conscious shopper's guide, which you will find beginning at page 233 of this book. In this we have listed many of the main carbohydrate-free or low-carbohydrate foods, and told you at what time of year to look out for them in the shops—when they are at their cheapest and at their best.

SLIMMER'S COOK BOOK

The recipes you will find beginning at page 207 can now also become your own, personal, Keep-Slim Cookery Book. Start to try out the ones which were part of other people's diets as well as the ones you are used to by now.

If you can choose your own, and your family's, meals from a long list of tasty dishes that are low in carbohydrate content, you are much less likely to get back again to cooking fattening meals.

It's a very good idea to add to this list of low-carbohydrate recipes yourself. By now you should have a very good idea of which foods are the fat-making culprits, and which aren't. Equip yourself with a notebook, and whenever you come across a recipe in a cookery book or magazine which is based mainly on protein and starch-free vegetable foods, jot it down.

You should be able to compile an impressive collection. And by turning to this book for your meal suggestions you'll help yourself stay slim.

DON'T LET THE POUNDS CREEP UP

It is still a matter of some importance that you should continue to make your weekly weight check (but not more often—remember?). If you don't own bathroom scales it's still worth dropping hints before your next birthday—even though you have now stopped your official slimming campaign.

In many ways it is now even *more* important to get weighed regularly. An extra stone or two of fat doesn't arrive in one large dollop; it creeps on gradually ounce by ounce. And as many of us who have sat on our major weight problem know

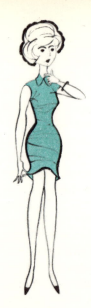

only too well, it's even sneaky enough to creep up behind.

Don't let an extra half stone or so surprise and dismay you in, say, six months' time. You can save yourself from having to initiate another major weight-losing campaign by tackling the pounds right away, if and when they come.

If you find that you have gained an extra 3 or 4 lbs., bring out your diet again. You can lose them in less than a fortnight.

We hope that you will have been able to buy some smart new clothes to set off your slim new figure. If so, resolve never again to "let out" your clothes to accommodate an expanding figure. Instead, "take in" your figure.

MAINTENANCE DIET

We have assumed that by the time you have lost the excess weight you had planned to lose you will want to stop your basic dieting.

But this isn't always the case. People vary enormously. Some can't wait to set fire to their diet sheet, while others tell us: "I think I shall carry on with my diet, I've got used to it."

If your appestat has become so well-trained that you don't want to stop following a diet then by all means carry on. This wouldn't be possible with "fad" diets, but with our methods it would be a healthy and easy procedure. It's the surest way of staying as slim as you are.

But for this purpose we would suggest that you follow a special maintenance diet which you can easily adjust to suit yourself from the method of Dieting by Numbers in this book—you will find it beginning on page 145.

This diet lends itself perfectly to stay-slim eating. It's a free-choice diet which lets you eat almost any food you like (though not necessarily all on the same day!) so it never becomes monotonous, however long you follow it.

When you study this method you will see that many of the foods are numbered and that for the dieting campaign we advise you to eat, in addition to "free foods", only those which add up to 12 or less in a day, if you want to lose weight.

On a maintenance diet, however, you can be more generous with yourself. To start with, try setting the number to 15.

If you find you are still losing a little weight—and you probably will—gradually set the number higher. You might well find the figure which perfectly balances the *status quo* somewhere in the 20's. When you find it, keep to it.

Now you aren't gaining, and you aren't losing. You have found out your own individual perfect maintenance diet, and you should find it very easy to follow. You are certainly going to be among the stay-slim winners!

KNOW YOUR ENEMIES!

If you belong to the "let's put the diet on the bonfire" school, your best stay-slim bet is to mark down your main enemies and just keep an eye on them.

Sugar is usually public enemy No. 1. With your re-trained appestat you may well find that now you can eat pretty well whatever you like, yet keep your weight down by consciously controlling only your intake of sweet foods.

It would be silly to go back to taking sugar in your tea if you are now getting used to drinking it unsweetened, or with sugar substitute, and now that you are out of the habit of eating chocolates and sweets, it would be a good idea to tell your family and friends that these things are now quite definitely off the gift list. Just let them know that

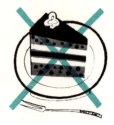

you don't fancy them any more—which is more than likely quite true!

Many families miss out the sweet course from their meals as a matter of habit—and wouldn't really want one if it was offered. By now you should have lost much of your craving for sweet things, and could easily follow their example. Some women we know have taken to substituting a tasty little hors d'oeuvre, to begin, instead of carbohydrate-filled sweets afterwards.

Bread is another enemy that needs watching. It is a big temptation because it is always there as an easy snack. But here our tips on shopping are your best safeguard.

Potatoes and pastas are the other most obvious enemies of your stay-slim campaign.

If you can control these four culprits, you should have no difficulty at all in keeping trim.

SECRETS OF SUCCESS

There are lots of final words of advice that we should like to give you about the importance of staying slim now that you have achieved your goal. But probably the most important of these are, quite simply, the reminder we'll give you: "Don't forget what it was like to be fat."

If you are tempted to "let things go" then just remember how demoralizing it was never to be able to feel really attractive when you did your absolute darndest to dress up for some special night out. Remember how those slim girls made you feel immense. And how shopping for any new clothes was always really hard work.

If you were very heavy, remember how you used to huff and puff, particularly going upstairs, and think how much better you feel now.

Don't destroy all those pictures of you at your worst. Keep at least one—you can laugh at it now—and bring it out from time to time as a salutary reminder.

Perhaps the last words in this part of the book ought to come "straight from the horse's mouth". Or, at least, from the mouth of a slim, smart woman who used to be a fat one.

She lost over 2 stone while she was dieting with us, and when, out of interest, we tracked her down again a year later she had lost another stone by continuing on her own.

She looked fabulous—hardly recognizable from the woman we first met. Now, three years after we first introduced her to dieting, she continues to be a slim, attractive woman and will undoubtedly never go back to being overweight.

This is what she told us:

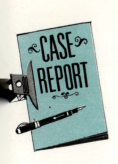

"I can't begin to describe the magic moments I have enjoyed since I became slim. Accidentally catching a sight of my new, slim silhouette in some shop window . . . dressing up for an evening out and liking the result . . .

People have asked me: 'But is being slim worth all the misery?'

And I reply: 'What misery?'

All I have given up are a few starchy foods, and what I've gained in return is tremendous energy, a wonderful sense of youth and well-being and new pride and pleasure in my appearance and the clothes I'm wearing.

In so many ways I am far happier slim than ever I was when I was fat.

As one of my many slimming bonuses, I have been able to take a big step forward in my career with a leading dress manufacturer. Now I am holding an interesting job which brings me into daily contact with many business clients. Frankly, I know I would never have been offered this if I was the same overweight woman I used to be.

Staying slim after a diet's over isn't hard; it takes just a little bit of will-power and common sense, for I can honestly say that at the end of my diet I had lost much of my previous craving for bread, potatoes and sweet things.

And I had learned such a lot.

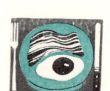

One of the things I learned is that a cooked breakfast makes slimming easier for the rest of the day. I don't become hungry after such a good start, so there's no temptation to nibble.

This is the basis of my eating now: I have almost completely cut out potatoes and sweet things like chocolate, cakes and puddings. I limit alcohol to just an occasional drink, and on most days I avoid bread.

What does this leave me with? Lots and lots of delicious meals that I really enjoy.

What could be more mouthwatering than a steak or mixed grill with mushrooms, tomatoes and green vegetables? Think of all the tasty fish dishes, the variety of tempting and inexpensive omelets you can enjoy. After a good meal like this I will often have cheese instead of pudding, or I might have a piece of fruit.

I drink my tea and coffee without sugar. It's surprising how quickly you get to like it much better that way.

Moments of temptation do come occasionally. During the weekdays when I go out to work I am never consciously aware of depriving myself. But at weekends I sometimes have to watch myself. To my great surprise I have found the strongest of allies in my teenage children who are quick to yell a warning if they see me wavering. They obviously much prefer to see me slim—as I am now.

I did have one slimming lapse when I was on holiday, because we were living in a caravan and tended to rely on snacks rather than cooked meals, so I gained 5 lbs. during those weeks. But I went right back on a diet when I came home and lost them in another two weeks.

The important thing is to make up for lapses right away before the extra weight and inches become demoralizing.

Because dieting has done so much for me I have become particularly interested in the subject and, on occasions when I have gained pounds, I have tried some different types of high-speed diets.

For almost a couple of weeks I once managed to stick to grapefruit and eggs alone—the diet that I picked up from a newspaper. That was very hard going; but I lost my few extra pounds very quickly. However, much to my dismay, I actually put on the weight again more quickly than I had taken it off when I went back to my normal eating.

The same thing happened when I tried a liquid diet. I had a most uncomfortable couple of weeks, lost weight quickly, then put it straight back on.

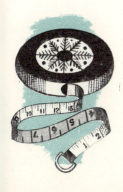

I have certainly proved conclusively to myself that the low carbohydrate type of diet works best of all in the long run. It may not always be quite as fast as some of the spartan diets, but for me it is the only diet that beats that "gone today, here tomorrow" problem.

I am not the only person in our family to whom slimming has meant almost a new life.

About a year and a half ago, my seventy-two year old mother, weighing 11 stone 4 lbs., consulted our family doctor about her health. She was suffering from arthritis and felt generally low with aches, pains and exhaustion.

The doctor recommended her to lose weight, so she asked me to show her how it was done.

Now she weighs 9 stone 6 lbs. and she really is a new woman. She tells everyone that she hasn't felt so fit for years.

The biggest bonus in figure-conscious eating is that the longer you do it the easier it gets. Temptation tends to fade away.

When you eat, and what you want to eat, I have discovered, depends very much on habit.

My new kind of eating has now become effortless and natural. I know that I shall never become fat again."

Well, we think that this lady has said it all. We wish you equal success!

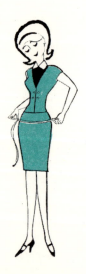

PART II

1. A loaded table for a good family tuck-in, but a WOMAN diet slimmer leaves rolls and scones for the others to polish off

2. Succulent and mouthwatering steak—there's no necessity to resist its temptation if you're following Rule of Three Diet

3. Cucumber Gala Salad (in the recipe section) will be popular if you're Dieting by Numbers—it's made up of "free" foods

4. When you "Choose Your Own Time" for eating, you'll find that Salade Niçoise is almost a complete meal in itself, any time

5. A Two-by-Two diet mixed salad, for Fruit and Vegetable days, can be presented so attractively that everyone will want some

6. There's no chance of going hungry on any WOMAN diet when there's so much to choose from, virtually carbohydrate-free

7. Orange Puffs with Vanilla Sauce provide a delectable finish to a meal when you're following the "Start-Right" diet plan

8. Chicken with Lemon Butter, only one of the many "Tempting Choice" dishes that will appeal to anyone who loves her food

9. Apple Cups, on the "Surprise Menu", look so pretty the family will clamour for them—luckily, they're so easy to prepare

10. Nothing could be simpler than the "Speedy Choice" of a bacon and egg breakfast—yet such an important start to the day

11. A "Simple Menu" for a packed lunch, but satisfying—and like all packed lunches we suggest, easily carried about with you

12. WOMAN diets let you lead as glamorous a life as you please; when a special date crops up, just Diet by Numbers that day

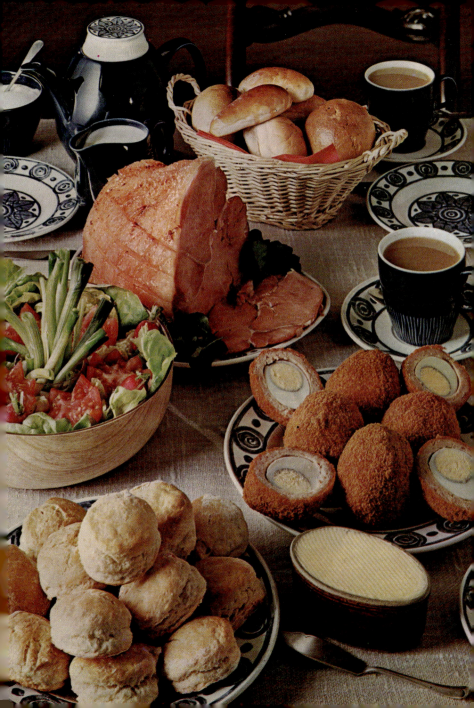

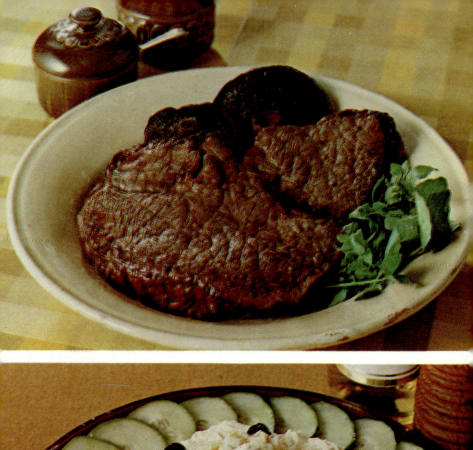
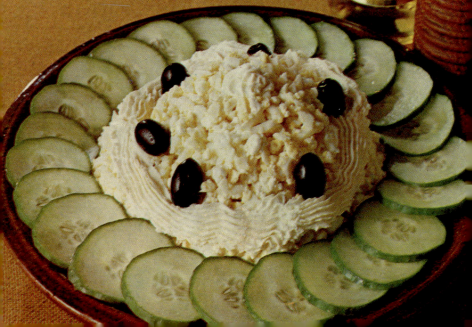

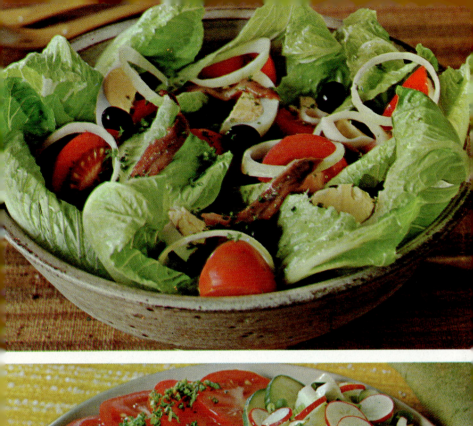
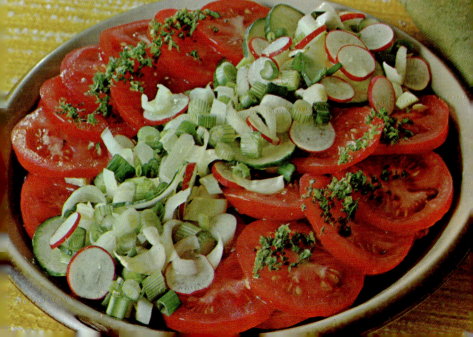

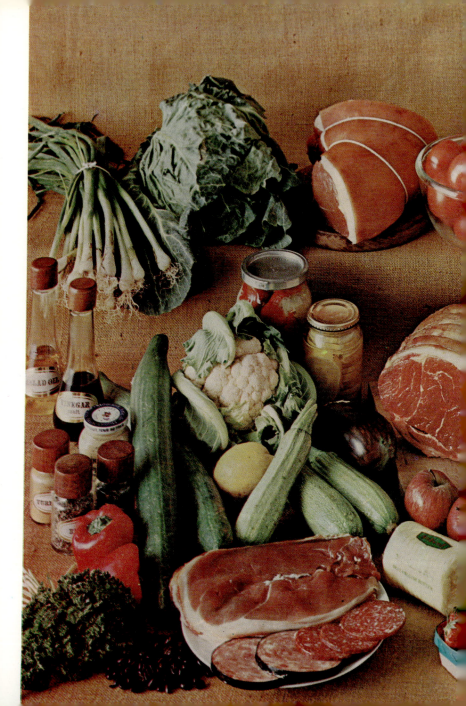

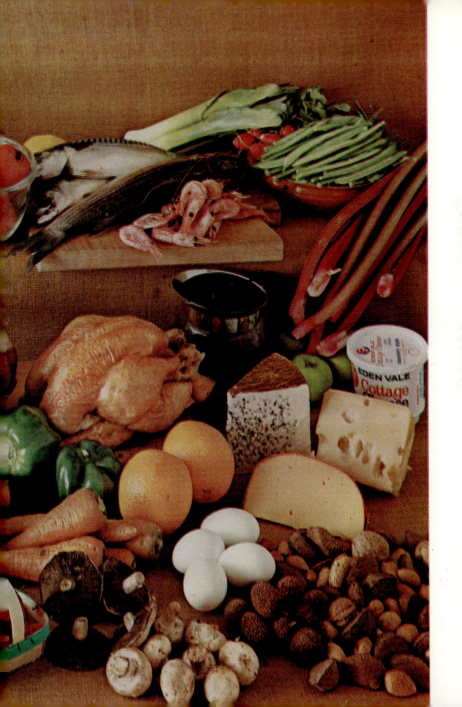

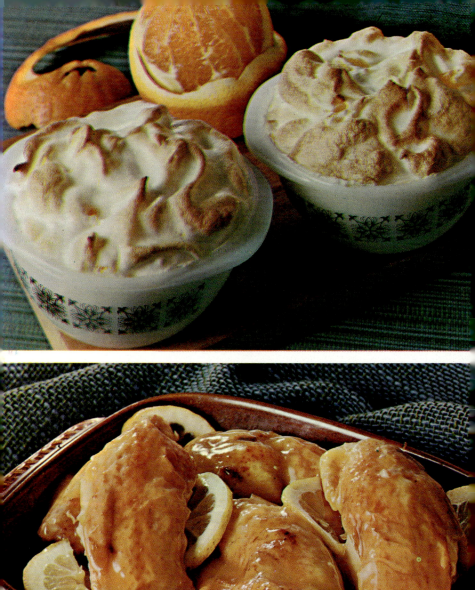
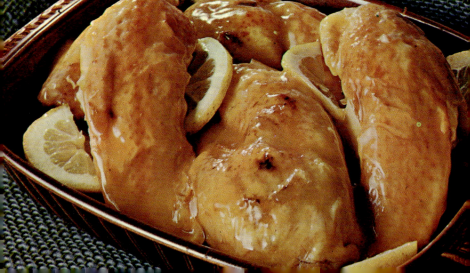

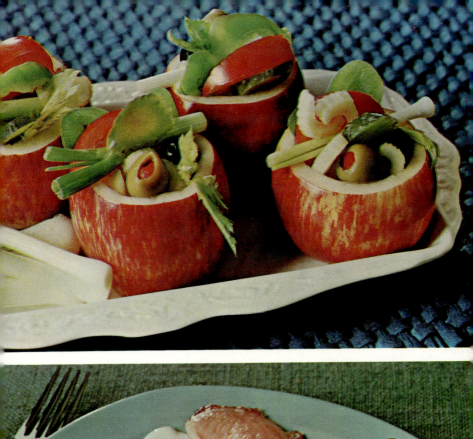

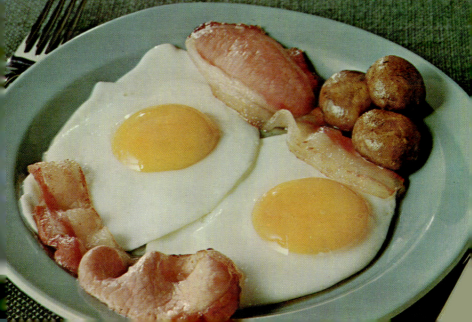

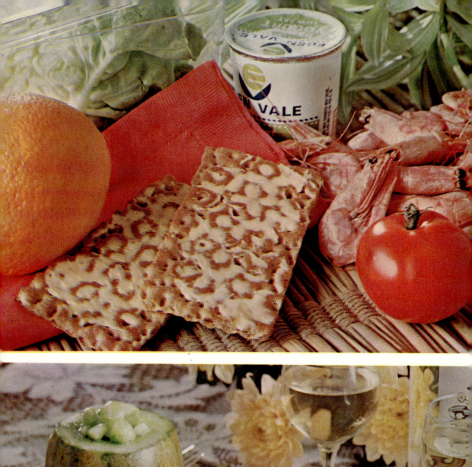
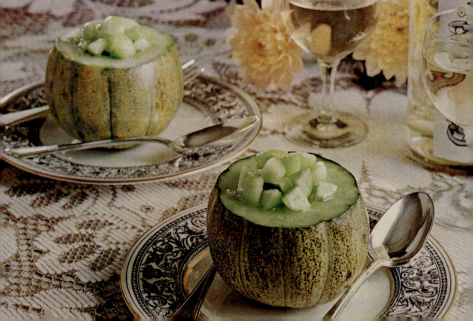

Woman

SPECIAL-DESIGN DIETS

THESE BASIC RULES apply to all WOMAN diets in this book and are an essential part of them—breaking the rules could spoil the effectiveness of any of the diets. Where any of the rules need to be slightly varied, or added to, the introduction to the particular diet will give you all the instructions you need.

1. Consult your doctor for permission to follow your diet unless you are absolutely certain that you are in perfect health.

2. Drink milk—half a pint each day in addition to each day's menus.

3. Drink as much as you like of water, tea, coffee, unsweetened lemon juice (including PLJ), sugar-free tonic water and sugar-free fruit drinks, and meat or vegetable extract drinks like Oxo, Bovril and Marmite. (Any milk you have in tea or coffee, etc., must be from your basic half pint; extra tea may be taken milkless with a slice of lemon.)

4. Sweeten drinks only with sugar substitutes in tablet and liquid form—Saxin, Sweetex, Hermesetas, Energen non-sugar sweetener, Bisks Sweetener, Sweetona, Minnim Cubes, Fullsweet, Sucron, Mini-Lumps.

5. Use sugar substitutes only (as above) in all cooking or sweetening.

6. Do not drink anything that is not listed above or specifically in your diet menu.

7. Eat as large a portion as you like of any of the foods on your diet menu, unless a set portion is particularly stated.

8. Choose starch-reduced products when crispbreads and rolls are listed on your menu. Crispbreads—Starch-Reduced Ryvita, Energen; rolls—Allinson, Energen and Granose. If you prefer the starch-reduced loaves to these products you may eat one thin slice of high-protein Cambridge Formula, or Top Diet, in place of each crispbread or roll.

9. Do not attempt to miss a meal, in particular a cooked breakfast.

ABBREVIATIONS USED IN THE DIETS AND RECIPES

av =	average
dspn =	dessertspoon
gl =	glass
hpd =	heaped
lb =	pound
lev =	level
lge =	large
med =	medium
oz =	ounce
pkt =	packet
pn =	portion
pt =	pint
sl =	slice
sm =	small
sug sub =	sugar substitute
swtd =	sweetened
tbspn =	tablespoon
tspn =	teaspoon

NOTE: When you want a packed lunch, remember how useful a vacuum flask is for clear soup or a hot drink; also the handy little plastic boxes with tight-fitting lids that are widely available, for "packing".

DIETS THAT LET YOU CHOOSE

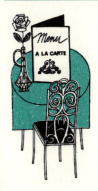

THESE DIETS are for the people who find it very important to be able to choose their own meals, and prove that this choosing can be done on a diet—even a fast one.

The first two diets give the widest possible element of free choice. The third gives a more limited choice, but some people will find it suits them best. To pin-point the right diet for you in this section, answer the questions at the beginning of each. If, after that, you are still not quite decided, try the questions above "Tempting Choice Diet" (page 171) and "Speedy Choice Diet" (page 184). These also give an element of choice and may suit some who regard choice as important, tied to other factors equally important to them.

Remember—the Basic Rules of WOMAN Diets (page 133) apply to all these diets.

RULE OF THREE DIET
average speed weight loss

Questions to ask yourself:
1. **Do I generally enjoy working things out for myself?**
2. **Am I happiest when I'm working at a steady, unhurried, unchanging speed?**

If you answer "yes" to these questions, this diet is right for you in every respect. It is your easiest and—in the long run—your fastest way to achieve a slim figure.

The Rule of Three diet gives that wide element of choice, allows you to work meals out for yourself, and proceeds at an even and unchanging pace. In fact it is the fastest "average-speed weight loss" diet in this book, but just not quite strict enough to rate in the next category.

The diet provides you with a see-at-a-glance dictionary of foods, split into three columns—it begins on the facing page.

Column One foods contain a moderate amount of carbohydrate and so must be carefully rationed. *Column Two foods* are low in carbohydrates, but still need to be limited, while *Column Three foods* are free of carbohydrate and can be eaten in any quantity.

Your diet takes care of all your rationing when you follow this simple method: Eat three or four meals each day. At each meal eat as much as you like from Column Three. But *during any one day* eat only 2 foods from Column One *or* 4 foods from Column Two.

If you prefer, you may have 1 food from Column One, plus 2 foods from Column Two as your daily allowance—results will be just the same. And it doesn't matter if you eat all your daily ration of limited foods at one meal, or prefer to divide it out through all the meals of the day.

Do make sure that you eat at least one good helping of meat, fish, eggs or cheese (all from Column Three) each day. And make sure also that you have at least one good helping of green vegetables (mostly from Column Three) each day. You may, of course, use the Special-Design recipes from the recipe section which begins at page 207 but, remember, some of the ingredients may have to be included in your "rationing" for the day.

COLUMN ONE	COLUMN TWO	COLUMN THREE
APPLE	APPLES	ANCHOVIES
dumpling (sm pn)	baked (1 av)	ASPARAGUS
pie (sm pn)	fresh (1 av)	ASPIC
pudding (sm pn)	stewed (av pn)	AUBERGINES
APRICOTS	with sug sub	
dried (2½ oz)	APRICOTS	
tart (av pn)	fresh (½ lb)	
ARTICHOKES	canned (¼ sm can)	
Jerusalem (sm pn)	ARTICHOKES	
	globe (2)	
BANANAS	BEANS	BACON
fresh (1 av)	broad (2 oz)	BEANS
fritters (1 sm)	BEETROOT	green
BARLEY	(1 lge)	BEEF
cooked (3 oz	BISCUITS	BEEFBURGERS
= 1 oz raw)	savoury (3 sm)	(Birds Eye)
BEANS	sweet (2 sm)	BRAINS
baked (2 tbspn)	BLACK-	BRAWN
butter (2 tspn)	CURRANTS	BUTTER
haricot (½ lb)	cooked (av pn)	
BEER	with sug sub	
(½ pt)	fresh (av pn)	
BLACK-	BLANCMANGE	
CURRANT	(av pn)	
purée (av pn)	BRANDY SNAPS	
BLACK	(1 sm)	
PUDDING	BRAZIL NUTS	
(av pn)	(4 oz)	
BREAD	BREAD	
and butter pudding	brown or	
(av pn)	white (1 sl)	
sauce (av pn)	crispbreads (2)	
BUNS	rolls, starch-	
1 (all types)	reduced (4)	

COLUMN ONE	COLUMN TWO	COLUMN THREE
	BROCCOLI ($\frac{1}{2}$ lb) BRUSSELS SPROUTS ($\frac{1}{2}$ lb) BUBBLE AND SQUEAK (av pn)	
CAKE plain (1 av sl) rich (1 sm sl) CHERRIES stewed (sm pn) canned ($\frac{1}{4}$ sm can) CIDER ($\frac{1}{3}$ pt) COCKTAILS (1 med gl) CORNISH PASTIES (1 lge) CUSTARD tart (sm pn)	CABBAGE raw (av pn) CARROTS (2 lge) CAULIFLOWER cheese (av pn) CHEESE sauce (av pn) straws (av pn) CHERRIES fresh ($\frac{1}{4}$ lb) glacé (8 av) CHICKEN patties (1) CHOCOLATE drink, $\frac{1}{2}$ milk $\frac{1}{2}$ water (1 cup) CHUTNEY (av pn) COCOA drink, $\frac{1}{2}$ milk $\frac{1}{2}$ water (1 cup) COCONUT desiccated (2 hpd dspn) CORNFLAKES (1 hpd tbspn)	CABBAGE boiled CAULIFLOWER boiled CELERY CHEESE CHICKEN boiled roast CHICORY COBNUTS COCKLES COFFEE black, sug sub CORNED BEEF CRAB CREAM CUCUMBER CURRY POWDER

COLUMN ONE	COLUMN TWO	COLUMN THREE
	CORNFLOUR ($\frac{1}{2}$ lev tbspn) COTTAGE PIE (av pn) CRUMPETS (1 av) CURRANTS dried (2 tbspn) CUSTARD (av pn)	
DAMSON tart (av pn) DOUGHNUTS (1 av) DUMPLING (1 av)	DAMSONS fresh ($\frac{1}{4}$ lb) canned ($\frac{1}{4}$ sm can) DATES (4 av)	DRIPPING DUCK
		EELS EGGS ENDIVE
FIGS dried (2 oz) FLOUR ($\frac{1}{2}$ oz) FRUIT DRINKS cordial ($\frac{1}{2}$ pt) squash ($\frac{1}{2}$ pt) fizzy ($\frac{1}{2}$ pt)	FISH cakes (1) fried (in batter) pie (av pn) FRANKFURTERS (4 lge) FRUIT DRINKS fresh juice (1 sm gl) FRUIT SALAD fresh (av pn) with sug sub canned (3 oz)	FIGS fresh FISH baked boiled fried (no batter) grilled poached paste roe FISH FINGERS

COLUMN ONE	COLUMN TWO	COLUMN THREE
GINGER ale ($\frac{1}{2}$ pt) beer ($\frac{1}{2}$ pt) bread (sm sl) GRAPES canned (av pn)	GOOSEBERRIES fresh ($\frac{1}{4}$ lb) stewed (av pn) canned (3 oz) GRAPEFRUIT fresh (1 lge) canned (av pn) GRAPES fresh (4 oz)	GALANTINE GAME GARLIC GELATINE GHERKINS GIBLETS GOOSE
HOTPOT Lancashire (av pn) vegetable (av pn)	HONEY (2 lev tspn)	HAM HAMBURGER HARE HAZELNUTS HEARTS
IRISH STEW (av pn)	ICE CREAM (2 oz)	
JELLY dessert (av pn) JUNKET ($\frac{1}{2}$ pt)	JAMS (1 lev dspn) JELLY preserve (1 dspn)	
		KIDNEYS

COLUMN ONE	COLUMN TWO	COLUMN THREE
LEMON meringue pie (av pn) **LENTILS** dried (2 oz)	**LEMON** curd (1 lev dspn)	**LAMB** **LARD** **LEEKS** **LEMON** fresh (1 lge) **LETTUCE** **LIVER** **LIVER SAUSAGE** **LOBSTER** **LOGANBERRIES** fresh stewed, sug sub
MACARONI cooked (3 oz = 1 oz raw) **MACAROONS** (1 lge) **MARMALADE** pudding (av pn) **MINCE** pies (1)	**MALTED DRINKS** $\frac{1}{2}$ milk, $\frac{1}{2}$ water (1 cup) **MARMALADE** (1 lev dspn) **MELON** fresh (1 sl) **MERINGUE** (1 av) **MILK** condensed, swtd (2 lev dspn) evaporated (2 tbspn) whole ($\frac{1}{2}$ pt) **MOUSSE** (av pn)	**MARGARINE** **MARROW** bone vegetable **MEAT EXTRACT** **MEAT PASTE** **MUSHROOMS** **MUSSELS** **MUSTARD** English or French and cress **MUTTON**
NECTARINES canned (4 oz) **NOODLES** 2 oz cooked (3 oz = 1 oz raw)		

COLUMN ONE	COLUMN TWO	COLUMN THREE
ORANGES canned (4 oz)	OATMEAL cooked (1 dspn) ORANGES fresh (1)	OIL OLIVES OMELETS using filling from column 3 ONIONS OXTAIL OYSTERS
PEACHES canned (2 halves) PEARS canned (2 halves) PINEAPPLE canned (1 sl) PLUMS stewed (av pn) canned (1 oz) POTATOES baked (1 lge) boiled (1 lge) crisps (1 pkt) fried (1 lge) mashed (av pn) roast (2 av) salad (av pn) PRUNES stewed ($\frac{1}{2}$ lb)	PANCAKES (1 av) PARSNIPS (1 av) PASTRY all kinds (1 oz) PEACHES fresh (1 med) PEARS fresh (1 med) PEAS dried (1 tbspn) fresh (2 tbspn) frozen (2 tbspn) canned (2 tbspn) PEASE PUDDING (av pn) PICKLES sweet (1 lev tbspn) PINEAPPLE fresh (2 sl) PLUMS fresh (4) PORRIDGE (av pn) POTATOES jacket (1 sm)	PARSLEY PEPPERS red and green PEANUT BUTTER PEANUTS PICKLES savoury PIGEON PORK PRAWNS

COLUMN ONE	COLUMN TWO	COLUMN THREE
RASPBERRIES frozen (av pn) canned (½ sm can) RAVIOLI (av pn) REDCURRANTS fresh (av pn) stewed (av pn) RICE pudding (av pn)	RAISINS (1 tbspn) RASPBERRIES fresh (4 tbspn) RICE plain cooked (1 tbspn) RISSOLES (2 av)	RABBIT RADISHES RHUBARB stewed, sug sub

SAGO
(av pn)
SCONES
drop or plain (1)
SEMOLINA
pudding (av pn)
SHORTBREAD
(1 med)
SPAGHETTI
cooked (3 oz
   = 1 oz raw)
SPIRITS
(1 sm tot)
STEAK AND
   KIDNEY
pie (av pn)
pudding (av pn)
STOUT
(½ pt)
STRAWBERRIES
canned (½ sm can)
frozen (av pn)
SULTANA
pudding (av pn)
SWEETS
(1 oz)
	SAUCES
	brown (2 tbspn)
	sweet (2 tbspn)
	white (2 tbspn)
	SAUSAGES
	beef or pork (2 sm)
	roll (1 sm)
	SCOTCH EGG
	(2 av)
	SEMOLINA
	uncooked (1 tbspn)
	SHEPHERD'S PIE
	(av pn)
	SOUPS
	cream or thick
	   (½ pt)
	STRAWBERRIES
	fresh (av pn)
	SUGAR
	(1 lev dspn)
	SULTANAS
	(1 hpd tbspn)
	SWEDES
	(1 av)
	SYRUP
	(1 lev dspn)
		SALAD
		dressing, oil
		and vinegar
		SALAMI
		SALMON
		fresh, smoked and
		   canned
		SARDINES
		in oil
		SCALLOPS
		SHRIMPS
		SOUPS
		clear
		SPINACH
		SPRING GREENS
		STEAK
		STEAKLETS
		(Birds Eye)
		STEAKBURGERS
		(Frood, Findus)
		SUET
		SWEETBREADS
		fried
		stewed

COLUMN ONE	COLUMN TWO	COLUMN THREE
TANGERINES canned (av pn) TOAD-IN-THE- HOLE (av pn) TRIFLE (av pn)	TANGERINES fresh (3) TAPIOCA uncooked (1 tbsp) TOMATOES fresh (2 lge) juice (1 gl) canned (1 sm can) TONIC WATER (1 med bottle) TREACLE (1 dspn) TURNIPS (2 av)	TEA no milk, sug sub TONGUE TRIPE TUNA FISH TURKEY TURNIP TOPS
VEAL and ham pie (av pn) VERMICELLI cooked (3 oz = 1 oz raw) VOL-AU-VENT (1 sm)	VEGETABLE JUICE (1 can V8)	VEAL fried roast stewed VEGETABLE EXTRACT VENISON VINEGAR
WAFFLES (1 med) WINES sweet (1 sm gl)	WELSH RAREBIT (av pn) WINES dry (1 gl)	WALNUTS WATERCRESS WHELKS WINKLES
YORKSHIRE PUDDING (av pn)		YEAST YOGHOURT (unflavoured)

DIETING BY NUMBERS
adjustable speed weight loss

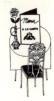

Questions to ask yourself:
1. **Do I generally enjoy working things out for myself?**
2. **Am I:**
   (a) A changeable person—often with more enthusiasm one week than another?
   (b) One who insists on fast results?

If you answer "yes" to the first question, and "yes" to either (a) or (b) in the second question this diet is the right one for you in every respect.

By "Dieting by Numbers" you can have a wide choice of food, work meals out for yourself by some simple calculations that you will probably enjoy, set your slimming pace as fast as you like, and even change the pace of your slimming when you feel like it.

The method is simplicity itself. By each of the alphabetically listed foods we have put a number. That number is directly related to the carbohydrate content of that food. The higher the number, the more carbohydrate the food contains, and therefore the stricter must be the rationing.

But on this diet you are allowed to eat as much as you like from a special list we give you of carbohydrate-free foods.

Don't forget your daily half pint of milk and the other **Basic Rules on page 133.**

Make sure you have at least one good helping of meat, fish or eggs daily, and at least one good helping of green vegetables.

You can, too, use the WOMAN Special-Design recipes which begin at page 207, but always remember to check the ingredients and include them in your daily count if they appear on your list of "numbered foods".

This is how to set the slimming speed that is right for you:

Do you want to set it really fast, and slim at top speed? Then eat three or four meals a day, helping yourself freely to foods on the carbo-hydrate-free food list.

For numbered foods, your daily numerical total is 5. That means, therefore, you can eat two or three foods where the numbers would add up to a daily total of 5.

This fast speed is, obviously, a rather strict diet, and so the importance of that additional half pint of milk must be emphasised. On no account miss it out.

Do you prefer to take it slowly—at least for a certain length of time?

Then the same rules apply, but the "total" you will choose is 12.

Many will find the slimming pace to suit their own will-power somewhere between these two extremes. In our experience, most people would be happiest around 9.

And of course it is quite easy to change in mid-stream, perhaps beginning with a low number to give you a good start when your enthusiasm is at its peak, then gradually increasing it towards 12 to finish at an easier pace. Or you could just as well change the number from week to week as your enthusiasm ebbs and flows.

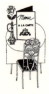

On the facing page you will see your list of "unrestricted foods". Eat as much as you like of them. On the following page begins your alpha-betical list of "numbered foods".

FOODS YOU CAN EAT FREELY

Meat of any description (including canned meat, bacon, poultry, offal, liver sausage)

Fish of any description (including canned fish, kippers, shellfish, eels, fish roes)

Cheese of any description (including processed cheese)

Butter, margarine, cream, *un*flavoured yoghourt, dripping, lard and oils (olive or salad); sour cream or unflavoured yoghourt may be used instead of mayonnaise

Eggs

Clear soups

These vegetables: asparagus, aubergines, cabbage, cauliflower, celery, chicory, cucumber, garlic, gherkin, green beans, lettuce, mushrooms, mustard and cress, olives, parsley, peppers, radishes, spinach, watercress

These nuts: almonds, brazil nuts, walnuts

These fruits: lemons, rhubarb (taking care to sweeten only with sugar substitute)

Aspic, curry powder, horse-radish, sour pickles, vinegar, salt

KEEP COUNT OF THESE FOODS

Do not exceed the daily number total between 5 and 12 that you have selected for your diet, when eating foods listed on these columns

A

ALMOND PASTE (1 oz) .... $\frac{1}{2}$
APPLE baked (sm) **2**
      dumpling (sm) **4**
      fresh (sm) **2**
      pie (sm pn) **6**
      stewed, no sugar (sm) ... **2**
APRICOT dried (2 oz) **4**
      fresh (med) **1**
      tinned (4 halves) **5**
ARTICHOKE **1**

B

BANANA............................. **5**
BARLEY (1 oz) **4**
BEANS baked (2 oz) **2**
      baked (on 1 sl toast)...... **5**
      broad (2 tbspn) fresh
      or frozen **2**
      haricot (2 tbspn) **3**
BEEFSTEAK AND KIDNEY
      pie (sm pn) **4**
      pudding (sm pn) :........ **4**

BEER mild (½ pt) **5**
      pale ale (½ pt) **5**
      stout (½ pt) **7**
      strong ale (½ pt) **6**
BEETROOT (small).................. **1**
BISCUITS savoury (3 sm) **3**
      sweet (2 sm) **3**
BLANCMANGE (sm pn) **2**
BREAD brown (thin sl)............ **3**
      crispbreads (2) **3**
      roll **6**
      starch reduced
      crispbread (1) **1**
      starch reduced
      rolls (2) **1**
      toast (thin sl) **3**
      white (thin sl) **3**
      wholemeal (thin sl) **3**
      and butter pudding
      (sm pn) **4**
BREAKFAST CEREALS
      All-bran (1 oz) **3**
      ordinary (2 tbspn) **4**
      starch reduced
      (2 tbspn) **3**
      sugar-coated
      (2 tbspn) **5**
BUN **5**

C

CAKE cream (2 oz pn) **6**
      plain (2 oz pn) **5**
      rich fruit iced
      (2 oz pn)..................... **8**
CANDIED PEEL (½ tbspn) **3**
CARROT (med) **1**
CASHEW NUTS (1 oz) **2**
CHERRIES fresh (¼ lb) **3**
      canned (¼ lb) **4**

CHESTNUTS (6) 3
CHICKEN PATTY 3
CHOCOLATE milk bar (1 oz)......$2\frac{1}{2}$
    plain bar (1 oz) ....$2\frac{1}{2}$
    powder (1 lev dspn) 1
CHRISTMAS PUDDING (sm pn) ... 8
CHUTNEY (lev dspn)............... 1
CIDER ($\frac{1}{2}$ pt) 7
COCKTAIL (sm gl)................. 4
COCOA powder (lev dspn) ...... $\frac{1}{2}$
COCONUT desiccated
    (2 hpd dspn) .... $\frac{1}{2}$
CORN ON COB (med)............... 4
CORNFLOUR (lev tbspn) ....$2\frac{1}{2}$
CORNISH PASTY (med) 4
COTTAGE PIE (sm pn) 3
CRANBERRIES fresh (2 oz) 1
    sauce (tbspn) 3
CRUMPETS (2) 3
CURRANTS dried
    (2 hpd tbspn) 3
    red (2 hpd tbspn) 1
CUSTARD (sm pn)................. 2

D

DAMSONS (4) 2
DATES (6) 4
DOUGHNUT 6
DUMPLING........................... 3

F

FIGS (4) 6
FISH CAKE 2
FISH PIE (sm pn) 2
FLOUR white or
    wholemeal (1 oz)......... 4

FRANKFURTER (lge) .... $\frac{1}{2}$
FRESH FRUIT SALAD (sm pn)...... 3
FRITTER apple 6
       banana 7
       pineapple ....$6\frac{1}{2}$
FRUIT DRINKS
       cordial, diluted ($\frac{1}{2}$ pt) ... 5
       lemonade ($\frac{1}{2}$ pt) 5
       pure juice (sm gl)......... 2
       pure juice, swtd
       (sm gl) 4
       squash, diluted ($\frac{1}{2}$ pt) ... 5

G

GINGER ALE ($\frac{1}{2}$ pt) ....$7\frac{1}{2}$
       beer ($\frac{1}{2}$ pt) ....$7\frac{1}{2}$
       dry ale ($\frac{1}{2}$ pt) 5
GINGERBREAD (sm sl) 6
GLACÉ CHERRIES (4) 1
GLUCOSE (lev tbspn) 6
GOOSEBERRIES (4 oz)............... 2
GRAPES (4 oz) 3
GREENGAGES (4) ....$2\frac{1}{2}$

H

HAZEL NUTS (15) .... $\frac{1}{2}$
HONEY (lev tbspn) 5
HOTPOT Lancashire (sm pn) ... 4
       vegetable (sm pn) 4

I

ICE CREAM (2 oz pn)............... 3

J

JAM (lev dspn) **3**
JELLY dessert (2 tbspn) **4**
      preserve (dspn) **3**
JUNKET (4 oz) **3**

L

LEEK .... $\frac{1}{2}$
LEMON ....**1$\frac{1}{2}$**
    and meringue pie
    (sm pn) **4**
LENTILS dried (2 oz)............... **6**
LOGANBERRIES (4 oz) **1**

M

MACARONI cheese (sm pn) **7**
    cooked (6 oz).........**10**
    uncooked (2 oz) ...**10**
MACAROON (sm) **3**
MALTED DRINKS (1 cup) **2**
MARMALADE (lev dspn) **3**
    pudding (sm pn) ... **5**
MELON (med sl)..................... **2**
MERINGUE ....**2$\frac{1}{2}$**
MILK condensed and swtd
    (2 lev tbspn) **3**
    evaporated (2 lev
    tbspn).................. $\frac{1}{2}$
    skimmed ($\frac{1}{2}$ pt) **3**
    whole ($\frac{1}{2}$ pt) **3**
MINCEMEAT (dspn) ....**3$\frac{1}{2}$**
MINCE PIE (sm) **4**
MOUSSE (2 oz pn) **2**

O

OATMEAL (tbspn) ....$3\frac{1}{2}$
ONION (med)......................... $\frac{1}{2}$
ORANGE (med) **2**

P

PANCAKE (sm) **2**
PARSNIP............................. **2**
PASTE fish (tspn) .... $\frac{1}{2}$
    meat (tspn) .... $\frac{1}{2}$
PASTRY (1 oz) **2**
PEACH fresh (med) **2**
    canned (2 halves) **5**
PEANUTS (30 nuts) **1**
    butter (1 oz) **1**
PEAR fresh (med).................. **2**
    canned (2 halves) ....$4\frac{1}{2}$
PEAS dried (2 tbspn)..............$3\frac{1}{2}$
    fresh or frozen
    (2 tbspn)..................... **2**
    canned garden and
    processed (2 tbspn) **2**
PEASE PUDDING..................... **3**
PICKLES sweet (lev dspn)......... **1**
PINEAPPLE fresh (3 sl) ....$2\frac{1}{2}$
    canned (3 sl) **8**
PLUMS fresh (2) **1**
    canned (4) **4**
PORRIDGE (sm pn) **3**
POTATO boiled (lge).............. **4**
    fried (lge) **4**
    mashed (lge) **4**
    roast (lge) **4**
    salad (lge) **4**
PRUNES dried ($\frac{1}{4}$ lb) **4**
    canned (4) **4**

R

RAISINS (2 hpd tbspn) 7
RASPBERRIES fresh (4 oz)......... 4
          canned (4 oz) 6
RAVIOLI cooked (6 oz)............10
          uncooked (2 oz).........10
RICE cooked (lev tbspn) 1
          uncooked (lev tbspn)... 5
RISSOLE 1
ROLY POLY PUDDING (sm pn)... 8

S

SAGO PUDDING (2 tbspn)......... 4
SAUCE brown (tbspn) 1
       sweet (tbspn) 1
       white (tbspn) .... $\frac{1}{2}$
SAUSAGES (1)......................$1\frac{1}{2}$
SCONE 5
SCOTCH EGG 2
SEMOLINA pudding (2 tbspn) ... 4
SHEPHERD'S PIE (sm pn) 3
SHORTBREAD (1 piece)............ 4
SORBITOL (lev tbspn) 6
SOUPS cream ($\frac{1}{2}$ pt) 2
      thick ($\frac{1}{2}$ pt) 2
SPAGHETTI cooked (6 oz) 10
     in tomato sauce
     (sm pn) 4
     uncooked (2 oz) 10
SPIRITS brandy (sm tot) 4
     gin (sm tot) 4
     rum (sm tot)............... 4
     whisky (sm tot) 4
SPONGE PUDDING (sm pn) 10
STRAWBERRIES fresh (4 oz) ......$1\frac{1}{2}$
     canned (4 oz) 2
SUET PUDDING (sm pn) 8
SUGAR brown and white
     (lev tspn) 1

SULTANAS (2 hpd tbspn) **4**
SWEDE **2**
SWEETS (1 oz) **5**
SYRUP (dspn) **2**

T

TANGERINES (3)..................... **2**
TAPIOCA pudding (2 tbspn)...... **5**
TOAD IN THE HOLE (sm pn) **5**
TOMATO fresh (lge) **1**
      juice ($\frac{1}{4}$ pt) **1**
      canned (2 med) **1**
TONIC WATER (sm bottle) ......**1$\frac{1}{2}$**
TREACLE (dspn) **2**
TRIFLE (sm pn)..................... **6**
TURNIP **1**

V

VEAL AND HAM PIE (sm pn)...... **6**

W

WAFFLE **4**
WELSH RAREBIT
      (on thin sl bread) **3**
WINE dry (lge wine gl)............ **3**
      port (lge wine gl) **6**
      sweet (lge wine gl)......... **4**

Y

YOGHOURT flavoured **4**
YORKSHIRE PUDDING (sm pn) ... **5**

CHOOSE YOUR OWN TIME DIET
average speed weight loss

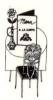

Questions to ask yourself:
1. **Do I often get stuck for ideas in planning meals?**
2. **Do I generally like "routine" and find it helpful?**
3. **Do I dislike calculations and prefer to have things worked out for me?**

If you answer "yes" to these questions you will find this diet ideal. To many, it will present the best of both worlds—an element of choice tied to the ease of routine.

WE choose the meals and present them to you already calculated and worked out.

YOU choose when you will eat each meal, because they are interchangeable.

This is how it works:

The diet is arranged as seven breakfasts, seven lunches, and seven evening meals, all interchangeable. As an alternative to a cooked lunch there are five interchangeable packed lunches for each week-day.

This means that *you choose*: twenty-one meals for the week in any order you like, provided only that you do not have the same meal twice in any one week.

You will probably prefer to have "breakfast" at breakfast time, but if you would like to have one of the evening meals at mid-day and vice-versa, it will not upset the diet.

To be certain you don't choose the same meal twice in one week it is a good idea to tick off each meal as it is eaten. Make sure your ticks are in pencil so that at the end of the week you can rub the letters out and won't be confused when you start again.

Basic WOMAN Diet Rules (page 133) apply, and starred recipes begin at page 207.

BREAKFASTS

1
Omelet, Bacon*, $\frac{1}{2}$ thin slice bread and butter

2
Boiled eggs, $\frac{1}{2}$ thin slice bread and butter

3
Fried bacon, $\frac{1}{2}$ thin slice bread and butter

4
Scrambled eggs, $\frac{1}{2}$ thin slice bread and butter

5
Ham and poached eggs, $\frac{1}{2}$ thin slice bread and butter

6
Grilled bacon, scrambled eggs, $\frac{1}{2}$ thin slice bread and butter

7
Bacon and eggs, $\frac{1}{2}$ thin slice bread and butter

LUNCHES

1
Minced meat OR braised beef, cauliflower OR green beans

2
Fish fried in egg and breadcrumbs, 1 tomato, 2 tbspn peas
Unflavoured yoghourt

3
Lamb OR pork chops, cabbage, 1 carrot, 2 tbspn rice pudding

4
Liver OR Meat Parcels*, green beans, 1 onion
4 stewed prunes OR 3 canned apricots

5
Hamburger* OR frozen Beefburgers OR Steaklets
1 carrot and 1 tomato, 1 baked apple OR Princess Soufflé*

6
Boiled Bacon OR braised hearts, 2 tbspn peas
2 tbspn fresh fruit salad OR Orange Puffs with Vanilla Sauce*

7
Meat OR poultry, Green Salad*, Saucy Pudding

PACKED LUNCHES

1
2 crispbreads and butter, fresh or frozen prawns OR shrimps
lettuce and 1 tomato, 1 apple

2
2 crispbreads and butter, cheese, celery, 1 tomato, 1 orange

3
2 crispbreads and butter, mashed sardines OR hard-boiled egg
1 tomato, 6 fresh grapes

4
2 crispbreads and butter, liver sausage OR luncheon meat
watercress and lettuce, 1 pear

5
2 crispbreads and butter, ham OR tongue, celery, 1 apple

(N.B. No packed lunches for the other two days—the weekend)

EVENING MEALS

1
1 slice melon, Cheesey Eggs*, 1 crispbread and butter

2
Clear soup, Welsh Rarebit* OR Kedgeree*, Unflavoured yoghourt

3
Omelet, Mushroom OR Spinach*, 1 tomato
2 crispbreads and butter with cheese

4
Ham OR tongue, 1 sm baked potato in jacket
OR 2 crispbreads and butter, Coffee Cream Chiffon*

5
Kippers OR herrings with Chicory and Caper salad*
1 crispbread and butter, 1 baked apple (remember—sug sub!)

6
Corned beef, 2 tbspn canned vegetable salad, Green Salad*
1 tomato, 1 crispbread and butter with cheese

7
1 pn Salade Niçoise*, 2 crispbreads with butter and cheese

FLYING-STARTERS DIETS

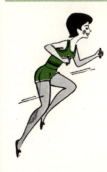

BOTH THE DIETS in this section are specially designed for the many people who are capable of showing strong diet determination, over a limited period of time.

They are strict diets and they are fast ones. They make the most of that initial spurt of enthusiasm. But by changing or easing the pace they give the necessary boost to will-power just when it is needed.

By frequent changes of eating pattern they also have a plus-factor in speeding up weight reduction. Our test-dieters have found them enormously effective. The first of these diets in particular, "Two-by-Two", has become something of a WOMAN classic.

TWO-BY-TWO DIET
high speed weight loss

Question to ask yourself:

Am I able to follow an unconventional pattern of eating without finding that it creates too many problems in my normal social, family or business life?

If the answer is "yes", if you can plan your eating to suit yourself without other considerations, then you are the one who can follow this highly effective WOMAN diet.

It gets you off to a flying start, and by continual changes of pattern keeps up a fast pace—and boosts your will-power.

The foods eaten are charted into groups of two days. First, two liquid days (which are the elimination days) in order to give you that flying start. These are followed by two protein days (when you eat mainly meat, fish, cheese and other protein foods). Then two mainly fruit and vegetable days.

After this you must alternate between the two protein days and two fruit and vegetable days for as long as you need to lose weight. The two liquid days are only to begin the diet and are not repeated.

The two-by-two rhythm, it's been found, really does speed up reduction: on no account must you switch the days around.

Because of this diet's special nature the **Basic WOMAN Diet Rules (page 133)** are slightly altered but only in these ways:

The daily milk allowance is increased on liquid days (see below). If hunger becomes a problem on fruit and vegetable days you are allowed to eat extra fresh fruits or salad vegetables (*not* potatoes) and you are also given a daily allowance of bread and butter or margarine.

Refer to the section beginning at page 207 for the starred recipes in your diet.

YOUR BASIC DAILY ALLOWANCE
(additional to each day's menu)

MILK:	1 pint on liquid days and fruit and vegetable days; ½ pint on protein days
BREAD:	8 Energen starch-reduced rolls, *or* 6 Energen starch-reduced crispbreads
BUTTER OR MARGARINE:	1 oz daily (you can check by cutting half a pound into eight equal portions)

2 LIQUID DAYS

FIRST DAY

BREAKFAST: 1 cup of tea *or* fresh orange juice
                Bread and butter from allowance

ELEVENSES: $\frac{1}{4}$ pint tomato juice

LUNCH: Clear soup *or* vegetable broth

TEA: 1 cup of tea (remember—milk from allowance!)

EVENING MEAL: Rest of milk allowance
                or Marmite vegetable extract drink
                Bread and butter from allowance

SECOND DAY

BREAKFAST: 1 cup of tea
                Bread and butter from allowance

ELEVENSES: $\frac{1}{2}$ pint fresh orange juice

LUNCH: Marmite vegetable extract drink

TEA: 1 cup of tea

EVENING MEAL: Rest of milk allowance *or* fresh orange juice
                Bread and butter from allowance

N.B. These two liquid (elimination) days occur only once, when you begin your diet course, and are not repeated.

2 PROTEIN DAYS

FIRST DAY

BREAKFAST: 1 cup of tea
2 tbspn starch-reduced breakfast flakes
Eggs, boiled, poached or cooked with butter from allowance *or* cold ham
Bread and butter from allowance

LUNCH: White fish *or* lean meat *or* grilled bacon
2 tbspn green beans
Unflavoured yoghourt *or* cheese
Bread from allowance

TEA: 1 cup of tea

EVENING MEAL: Meat *or* ham *or* white fish
or Baked Eggs with Cheese*
Small portion baked egg custard *or* junket
with 1 tspn honey

SECOND DAY

BREAKFAST: 1 cup of tea
2 tbspn starch-reduced breakfast flakes
White fish *or* bacon
Bread and butter from allowance

LUNCH: Meat *or* poultry *or* white fish
or 2 poached eggs and cheese
Small portion junket *or* unflavoured yoghourt
with 1 tspn honey

TEA: 1 cup of tea

EVENING MEAL: Clear soup *or* Bovril *or* Marmite extract drink
Meat *or* ham with 1 poached egg
or Omelet, Ham *or* Cheese*
Small portion junket *or* cheese
Bread from allowance

2 FRUIT AND VEGETABLE DAYS

FIRST DAY

BREAKFAST: 1 grapefruit *or* 2 oranges
1 cup of tea
Bread and butter from allowance
1 tspn honey

LUNCH: Clear soup *or* Marmite extract drink
Mixed Salad*
Fresh or stewed fruit with 1 dspn raisins

TEA: 1 cup of tea

EVENING MEAL: Tomato juice
Vegetable Stew with Tomato or Marmite gravy*
1 apple and 1 pear
or canned *or* bottled fruit drained of syrup,
with orange juice added

Rest of milk allowance at bedtime

SECOND DAY

BREAKFAST: 1 apple *or* 1 pear
4 stewed prunes *or* 1 banana
1 cup of tea
Bread and butter from allowance

LUNCH: Orange juice *or* clear soup
Mixed Salad* *or* Vegetable Plate*
Fresh or stewed fruit

TEA: 1 cup of tea

EVENING MEAL: Clear vegetable soup *or* Marmite extract drink
or tomato juice *or* fresh celery
French Cabbage* *or* Vegetable Plate* *or* Mixed
Salad*
Junket *or* jellied fresh fruit juice (use 1 tspn gelatine to $\frac{1}{3}$ pint juice)

Rest of milk allowance at bedtime

START-RIGHT DIET
high speed weight loss

Question to ask yourself:

Can I follow an unconventional pattern of eating —for limited periods only?

If you answer "yes" to this question because you feel that your diet really must allow a certain amount of "social, everyday eating" you will find that this diet hits on a very happy compromise.

It combines the flying start, and the plus factor of changing eating patterns, with a basis of normal everyday eating.

In this diet the "flying start" comes right at the beginning of each week, so that the unconventional eating pattern lasts for only two days of the week.

On Mondays and Tuesdays the menus are more restricted than those for the other days of the week. Monday menus are almost entirely liquid, and Tuesday menus are mainly fruit and vegetables. But for the remainder of the week you will find the menus are varied and give near-to-normal eating, limiting only the amount of carbohydrate you eat.

Basic WOMAN Diet Rules (page 133) apply, but on Mondays and Tuesdays drink *one pint* of milk, instead of the usual half pint.

You may, if you like, "swap" some of the meals *within the same day*—by eating your evening meal at mid-day and the "lunch" at night, say. You may, except on Mondays and Tuesdays, exchange any of the *breakfasts* for one listed for a different day, but this does *not* apply to the other meals.

You will find the recipes for your starred dishes in the section beginning at page 207.

MONDAY

BREAKFAST:	1 cup fresh orange juice 1 crispbread and butter Tea *or* coffee
ELEVENSES:	$\frac{1}{2}$ pint milk, with coffee if preferred
LUNCH:	Marmite *or* similar drink 1 crispbread and butter
PACKED LUNCH:	As for lunch
TEA:	Tea
EVENING MEAL:	Clear soup (made with bouillon cube or consommé) 1 crispbread and butter
BEDTIME:	Rest of 1 pint milk allowance *or* unsweetened lemon juice with hot water

TUESDAY

BREAKFAST:	$\frac{1}{2}$ grapefruit, 4 stewed prunes 1 crispbread and butter Tea or coffee
ELEVENSES:	$\frac{1}{2}$ pint milk, with coffee
LUNCH:	Clear soup or canned vegetable juice (V8) 1 crispbread and butter
PACKED LUNCH:	Mixed salad of tomato, lettuce cucumber, celery, watercress 1 pear
TEA:	Tea
EVENING MEAL:	Cauliflower Savoury* Stewed apple or Rhubarb Fool*
BEDTIME:	Rest of 1 pint milk allowance or Marmite drink

WEDNESDAY

BREAKFAST: Bacon and eggs
            $\frac{1}{2}$ thin slice bread and butter

LUNCH: Grilled steak *or* veal
            or Steaklets *or* Beefburgers
            1 onion
            cauliflower
            3 canned plums
            or Princess Soufflé

PACKED LUNCH: 2 crispbreads and butter
               liver sausage *or* ham
               watercress and celery
               1 pear

EVENING MEAL: Corned beef *or* tongue
               1 medium potato baked in
               jacket with butter
               or 2 crispbreads and butter

BEDTIME: Rest of $\frac{1}{2}$ pint milk allowance

THURSDAY

BREAKFAST: Omelet, Ham*
$\frac{1}{2}$ thin slice bread and butter

LUNCH: Liver and bacon
mushrooms
$\frac{1}{4}$ lb. runner beans
2 tbspn rice pudding

PACKED LUNCH: 2 crispbreads and butter
cheese
celery
1 tomato
1 orange

EVENING MEAL: Lamb chop
or salmon
or tuna fish
Green Salad*
2 crispbreads and butter

BEDTIME: Rest of $\frac{1}{2}$ pint milk allowance

FRIDAY

BREAKFAST: Scrambled eggs
$\frac{1}{2}$ thin slice bread and butter

LUNCH: Fish (fried in egg and breadcrumbs) *or* fish fingers
cauliflower
1 tomato
stewed apple

PACKED LUNCH: 2 crispbreads and butter
fresh or frozen prawns *or*
shrimps
lettuce and 1 tomato
1 apple

EVENING MEAL: Cream cheese and cucumber
or Cucumber Gala Platter*
celery
1 thin slice bread and butter

BEDTIME: Rest of $\frac{1}{2}$ pint milk allowance

SATURDAY

BREAKFAST: Bacon and eggs
$\frac{1}{2}$ thin slice bread and butter

LUNCH: Lamb chop *or* pork chop
Green Salad*
1 tomato
4 stewed prunes *or* Prune
Mousse*

EVENING MEAL: Stuffed Marrow*
or Stuffed Pepper*
1 crispbread and butter
1 orange

BEDTIME: Rest of $\frac{1}{2}$ pint milk allowance

SUNDAY

BREAKFAST: Grilled Grapefruit*
Omelet, Mushroom*

LUNCH: Spiced Breast of Lamb*
or poultry
5 brussels sprouts
2 tbspn jelly with
fresh cream *or* Orange Puffs
with Vanilla Sauce*

EVENING MEAL: Cream cheese
4 segments of orange
watercress
1 crispbread and butter

BEDTIME: Rest of $\frac{1}{2}$ pint milk allowance

FOOD-LOVERS' DIETS

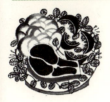

THESE ARE specially tasty and generous diets, allowing slimmers "a little of what they long for" now and then. You'll find here foods which are not normally associated with diets—apple dumplings, meringues, fish and chips. These foods are carefully calculated and allocated so they do not interfere with weight loss.

Although these diets aren't among the fastest in the book they are often the fastest in the long run for the woman who is used to hearty eating, the diets she will enjoy, and keep to, and with which she will succeed.

TEMPTING CHOICE DIET
average speed weight loss

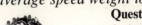

Questions to ask yourself:
1. Am I a comfort lover who often prefers the easiest possible path to success?
2. Do I find set routine rather tedious?

If you answer "yes" to both these questions this diet is right for you in every way. It is probably the easiest effective diet you will ever come across, and beats any fear of boredom by allowing a wide choice of meals.

Following this diet is simplicity itself. You have a list of breakfasts, lunches and of evening meals. Choose one of each, each day.

Timing of meals doesn't matter. You may eat a "lunch" in the evening, an "evening meal" at mid-day if you wish. But pick one of each. Don't choose, say, two lunches in one day.

Basic WOMAN Diet Rules (page 133) apply, and starred recipes begin at page 207.

BREAKFASTS

1. 2 tbspn porridge (milk from allowance, sug sub if required)
2 boiled eggs

2. 1 glass orange juice (made from 1 fresh orange)
Grilled gammon and 1 tomato

3. 1 glass unsweetened Pure Lemon Juice and water
Smoked haddock poached in milk, 1 thin slice toast and butter

4. Potted minced chicken with mushrooms
on 1 thin slice buttered toast

5. Bacon and egg
2 crispbreads and butter with 1 tspn jam *or* marmalade

6. 1 glass unsweetened Pure Lemon Juice and water
Poached egg on 1 thin slice buttered toast

7. Kidneys on 1 thin slice buttered toast

8. 1 glass unsweetened Pure Lemon Juice and water
Boiled eggs, 1 thin slice bread and butter

9. 1 glass unsweetened Pure Lemon Juice and water
Bacon and 3 tbspn baked beans

10. 1 glass unsweetened Pure Lemon Juice and water
4 tbspn stewed gooseberries, Bacon and 1 grilled tomato

11. Grilled chicken liver on 1 slice buttered toast

12. Grilled ham and mushrooms, 1 crispbread and butter, 1 apple

13. 2 tbspn starch-reduced cornflakes (use milk from allowance, sug
sub if required), Kippers

14. ½ grapefruit (use sug sub if required)
3 chipolata sausages with mushrooms, 1 tomato

15. 1 glass unsweetened Pure Lemon Juice and water
2 grilled Steakburgers, 1 thin slice toast and butter

16. 1 cold baked apple, Grilled kidney, bacon and 1 tomato

17. 1 glass unsweetened Pure Lemon Juice and water
Roes on 1 thin slice buttered toast

18. Grilled Grapefruit*, Cold ham

19. Haddock and scrambled eggs, 1 thin slice toast and butter

20. 2 tbspn starch-reduced cereal (milk from allowance, sug sub if required), Kidneys and bacon

21. 1 can V8 Vegetable Juice, Bacon, egg, 2 tbspn baked beans

22. 1 glass unsweetened Pure Lemon Juice and water
2 tbspn starch-reduced cereal (milk from allowance, sug sub if required), Bacon and fried cabbage

23. Scrambled eggs and shrimps, 1 thin slice toast and butter

24. 1 glass unsweetened Pure Lemon Juice and water, 2 fish cakes

LUNCHES

1. Grilled cod with 1 grilled tomato
1 crispbread and butter with cream cheese, 1 orange

2. Eggs on spinach, 1 small apple dumpling

3. Lettuce and cucumber salad
4 oz raspberries *or* 3 oz ice-cream

4. Cream soup, Grilled herrings, 2 crispbreads and butter

5. Luncheon meat with 1 lev dspn sweet pickle, Green Salad*
1 tomato, Cheese, 2 crispbreads and butter

6. Cold fresh or canned salmon, Lettuce and 2 tomatoes with
cucumber and radishes, 2 oz frozen mousse

7. Kippers, 2 hpd tbspn blancmange with fresh cream

8. Curried chicken, 4 tbspn cooked rice, Unflavoured yoghourt

9. Omelet, Tomato* with watercress
1 crispbread and butter, 1 apple *or* pear

10. Omelet, Spinach*, 2 crispbreads and butter with cheese
1 fresh peach

11. Meat Parcels*, Unflavoured yoghourt

12. Roast lamb, 1 medium potato and cabbage, Rhubarb Fool*

13. 2 Scotch Eggs*, Lettuce, spring onions and radishes
Unflavoured yoghourt

14. Cauliflower Au Gratin*, 2 tbspn blancmange and 1 tspn jam

15. Cheese Sandwich Soufflé*, Chopped raw cabbage
Unflavoured yoghourt

16. Clear soup, 2 large frankfurters, 2 tbspn baked beans
2 fresh apricots

17. Boiled beef and 2 tbspn pease pudding, 1 carrot and spinach
Unflavoured yoghourt

18. Cream soup, Cheesey Eggs*

19. 1 cup Bovril, Cold chicken, Lettuce, radishes and celery
1½ slices canned pineapple, Unflavoured yoghourt

20. Braised hearts, swede and 2 braised leeks
Unflavoured yoghourt topped with chopped walnuts
Cream cheese with 1 crispbread and butter

21. Stewed eels, 1 medium potato creamed with butter

22. Cream soup, Roast chicken, braised celery and broccoli
Prune Mousse*

23. Cream cheese with chopped green pepper and chives
Pink salad (1 cooked beetroot, 1 chopped onion, shredded raw
white cabbage), 1 small meringue with fresh cream

24. Buck Rarebit*, Green Salad*, 1 fresh apricot *or* tangerine

EVENING MEALS

1. Clear soup, Stuffed Peppers*, Flavoured yoghourt

2. Clear soup, Liver and bacon, cauliflower and cabbage
4 halves canned apricots with fresh cream

3. Clear soup, Roast chicken and 1 chipolata
brussels sprouts and 1 large roast potato

4. Pork chops, broad beans and mushrooms, 2 oz ice-cream

5. Cream soup, Casseroled steak, kidney and mushrooms
cabbage and green beans, 3 oz canned cherries

6. Roast beef, 1 potato baked in jacket, 3 stewed plums

7. Casseroled chicken, braised celery and 1 baked tomato
3 tbspn fruit salad with fresh cream

8. Braised steak, cauliflower and green beans
1 stewed apple and 2 oz ice-cream

9. Stuffed Marrow*, 1 banana

10. Cream soup, Danish Meat Balls*, Cauliflower and 2 carrots
Unflavoured yoghourt

11. Lamb chops, broccoli and 2 grilled tomatoes
3 canned plums with fresh cream

12. Cream soup, Cold salmon and Green salad*, Omelet, Sweet*

13. Grilled steak, 2 grilled tomatoes and 3 tbspn peas, Coffee Sponge*

14. Stewed beef, turnips, 1 carrot and cabbage, 4 oz grapes

15. Braised lamb, brussels sprouts and broad beans
1 apple *or* 1 fresh peach

16. Grilled veal with heated canned asparagus, courgettes
green beans and 1 tomato, Flavoured yoghourt

17. Cream soup, Kebabs*, 1 crispbread and butter with cheese

18. Grilled cod, 2 tbspn peas, Rhubarb Fool*
Cream cheese, 2 cream crackers

19. Liver and bacon with 1 fried onion, 2 tbspn peas
2 halves canned apricots with fresh cream

20. Cod en Cocotte*, 3 canned plums *or* 4 oz frozen mousse

21. Golden Hot Pot*, cauliflower and broad beans, 1 apple

22. Cold meat, mustard and cress, celery, 2 halves canned peaches
or 4 halves canned apricots, with fresh cream

23. Roast spare ribs of pork with small portion apple sauce mushrooms, cauliflower, 3 canned plums *or* 2 cream crackers and butter with cheese

24. Grilled pork chops with Mushroom Sauce*, broad beans marrow, 2 oz ice-cream

---

**ARE YOU REMEMBERING TO REFER
TO THE BASIC RULES, PAGE 133?**

average-quick speed weight loss

Questions to ask yourself:

1. Will I sacrifice just a little ease for a little more speed?

2. Do I generally like a set routine?

Those who answer "yes" will find this diet ideal; a fraction more restricted than the "Tempting Choice" one, it gives rather faster results but is still tasty and generous.

The repeating weekly pattern of a set menu tends to make shopping and planning easier.

Basic WOMAN Diet Rules (page 133) apply, and the starred recipes begin at page 207.

MONDAY

BREAKFAST
Bacon and eggs, 1 crispbread and butter

COOKED LUNCH
Mixed grill (chops, liver, kidney, etc., but *no* tomato), 1 tbspn peas, 1 carrot
2 tbspn jelly with fresh cream

PACKED LUNCH
Scotch Egg*, Green Salad* (no dressing)
2 crispbreads and butter
Unflavoured yoghourt, 1 small apple

EVENING MEAL
Clear soup, fish fingers, 1 grilled tomato
1 crispbread and butter with cheese

Rest of ½ pint milk allowance at bedtime

TUESDAY

BREAKFAST

Bacon and eggs
1 crispbread and butter

COOKED LUNCH

Grilled sausages, 2 tomatoes
2 slices pineapple with fresh cream

PACKED LUNCH

2 crispbreads and butter
2 cold sausages
celery *or* shredded cabbage
1 pear
cheese

EVENING MEAL

Liver pâté *or* luncheon meat
hard-boiled egg
Chicory and Caper Salad*
watercress, radishes
1 crispbread and butter

Rest of $\frac{1}{2}$ pint milk allowance at bedtime

WEDNESDAY

BREAKFAST

Bacon and eggs
2 crispbreads and butter

COOKED LUNCH

Liver
French Cabbage* (made with only 1 onion)
Coffee Sponge*

PACKED LUNCH

2 crispbreads and butter
fresh or frozen prawns
watercress
1 apple *or* 1 small peach
cheese

EVENING MEAL

Cauliflower Au Gratin*
grilled ham
1 crispbread and butter
Unflavoured yoghourt

Rest of $\frac{1}{2}$ pint milk allowance at bedtime

THURSDAY

BREAKFAST

Bacon and eggs
1 crispbread and butter

COOKED LUNCH

Braised hearts and mushrooms
5 brussels sprouts
Saucy Pudding*

PACKED LUNCH

1 crispbread and butter
cheese
1 tomato
celery *or* shredded cabbage
2 sweet biscuits

EVENING MEAL

Clear soup
Omelet, Tomato*
2 crispbreads and butter
Unflavoured yoghourt *or* Coffee Cream Chiffon*

Rest of ½ pint milk allowance at bedtime

FRIDAY

BREAKFAST

Boiled eggs
1 crispbread and butter

COOKED LUNCH

Fried fish with average portion chips
Unflavoured yoghourt

PACKED LUNCH

Small portion veal and ham pie
or cream cheese and 2 crispbreads and butter
Chicory
Watercress
1 apple
or 1 tangerine

EVENING MEAL

Clear soup
Sliced braised beef
or kippers
carrots
brussels sprouts

Rest of $\frac{1}{2}$ pint milk allowance at bedtime

SATURDAY

BREAKFAST
Bacon and eggs, 1 crispbread and butter

COOKED LUNCH
Grilled steak *or* escalop of veal
buttered cabbage, 2 tbspn trifle

EVENING MEAL
Clear soup, Supper Salad*
1 crispbread and butter

Rest of ½ pint milk allowance at bedtime

SUNDAY

BREAKFAST
Bacon and eggs, 1 crispbread and butter

COOKED LUNCH
Meat *or* Chicken with Lemon Butter*
cauliflower, 2 tbspn runner beans
Apricot Airy Fairy*

EVENING MEAL
Clear soup, Apple Cup*
Unflavoured yoghourt *or* Coffee Cream Chiffon*

Rest of ½ pint milk allowance at bedtime

SWIFT-AND-STRAIGHTFORWARD DIETS

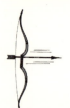

THESE DIETS have the joint virtues of being swift and being very simple. The meals are all carefully worked out for you on a basis of normal everyday eating. They could fit in particularly easily with ordinary family eating and would also be obtainable from the menus of most restaurants.

SPEEDY CHOICE DIET
high speed weight loss

Question to ask yourself:

Would I find an element of choice in eating helpful in a diet?

If you would this is the diet for you—combining speed, simplicity and choice.

Beginning on the next page, you are given a list of breakfasts, a list of lunches, and a list of evening meals. You can choose any one of each, each day.

Timing of the meals does not matter. You may eat a "lunch" in the evening and an "evening meal" at lunchtime if you wish. But pick one of each. Don't have, for instance, two lunches in one day.

Refer to the Basic WOMAN Diet Rules on page 133 and the Special-Design recipes for your starred dishes, starting at page 207.

BREAKFASTS

1. Kippers, 1 crispbread and butter

2. Bacon and egg, 1 crispbread and butter

3. Boiled eggs, 1 crispbread and butter

4. Scrambled eggs, 1 crispbread and butter

5. Bacon, 1 grilled tomato

6. Grilled kidney and bacon, 1 crispbread and butter

7. Smoked haddock poached in milk, 1 crispbread and butter

8. Bacon and mushrooms, 1 crispbread and butter

9. Poached eggs, 1 sausage

10. 1 can V8 Vegetable Juice, Cold boiled ham

11. Bacon and egg, 1 tomato

12. Omelet, Bacon or Cheese*, 1 crispbread and butter

13. Scrambled eggs, chopped shrimps, 1 crispbread and butter

14. Kidney and mushrooms, 1 crispbread and butter

15. 4 frankfurters, 1 small tomato (hot or cold)

16. $\frac{1}{2}$ grapefruit, Tomato Special*

17. Liver and bacon, 1 crispbread and butter

18. Bloaters, 1 crispbread and butter

19. Kedgeree*

20. Grilled herrings, 1 crispbread and butter

21. Grilled Grapefruit*, Boiled egg, 1 crispbread and butter

22. Liver, 1 small sausage

23. Grilled ham, poached eggs, 1 crispbread and butter

24. Stewed rhubarb, cold ham, 1 crispbread and butter

LUNCHES

1. Maximilienne Eggs*, grilled bacon

2. Plaice OR cod, topped with grated cheese and grilled

3. 2 Hamburgers*, OR frozen Beefburgers, 2 tbspn peas
   Unflavoured yoghourt

4. 2 fish cakes, green beans, Unflavoured yoghourt

5. Plain omelet, Green Salad*, 1 apple OR 1 orange

6. Hard-boiled eggs, cheese, watercress, radishes
   1 slice melon OR 3 oz grapes

7. Omelet, Ham*, 1 grilled tomato, 1 crispbread and butter

8. Fresh or frozen braised beef, 2 carrots, cabbage
   Unflavoured yoghourt

9. Corned beef OR any canned meat, watercress, lettuce, chicory
   1 orange

10. 2 poached eggs on spinach, Cheese, 2 crispbreads and butter

11. Fresh or frozen fillets of sole, spinach
    2 oz frozen mousse OR Prune Mousse*

12. Clear soup, sardines (canned in oil), mixed salad using 1 sm beetroot,
    watercress, cucumber, Unflavoured yoghourt

13. Roast veal, spinach, green beans, 2 oz frozen mousse

14. Omelet, Cheese*, green beans, 1 orange

15. Clear soup, Roast pork with gravy
    cauliflower, brussels sprouts
    1 baked apple with fresh cream

16. Jellied veal, cheese, gherkins, celery
    Unflavoured yoghourt, 1 fresh peach

17. Ham and Egg Humpies*, 1 apple

18. Roast beef with horseradish sauce, cauliflower, 2 leeks
    Cheese, 1 crispbread and butter

19. 2 frankfurters, 1 tomato, cole slaw
    1 crispbread and butter
    Unflavoured yoghourt OR Coffee Cream Chiffon*

20. Stewed steak, cabbage, cauliflower, 1 apple OR pear

21. Fried mackerel, Green Salad*, 4 tbspn stewed gooseberries

22. Tuna fish, Green Salad*, 1 small beetroot, 1 tomato
    Coffee Cream Chiffon*

23. Haddock topped with grated cheese, 1 slice melon OR 1 apple

24. Liver pâté, Chicory and Caper Salad*
    Cheese, 2 crispbreads and butter

EVENING MEALS

1. Clear soup, 2 grilled lamb chops, green beans, 1 carrot
   1 apple OR pear

2. Escalop of Veal with Cheese*, broccoli and green beans
   3 canned plums with fresh cream

3. Clear soup, Mixed grill
   (use steak, bacon, 1 sausage, kidney, liver, 1 tomato, 1 onion)
   1 portion Coffee Sponge*

4. Clear soup, Hawaiian Circle*, Unflavoured yoghourt

5. Fried chicken with Mushroom sauce*
   2 tbspn gooseberries (sug sub if required) with fresh cream

6. Braised liver and onion, cabbage, broccoli, Rhubarb Fool*

7. Cauliflower Au Gratin*, Unflavoured yoghourt

8. Clear soup, fish fingers, 2 tbspn peas, 1 small orange

9. Clear soup, Grilled ham steak, 1 grilled tomato
   1 baked apple with fresh cream

10. Stewed steak, kidney and mushrooms, brussels sprouts
    1 small potato, Rhubarb Fool*

11. Escalop of Veal with Cheese*, cauliflower, 4 oz grapes

12. Pork chop, cabbage, green beans, Quickie Pear*

13. Clear soup, Stuffed Peppers* OR Stuffed Marrow*

14. Beef (minced with 2 onions), cauliflower, spinach
    2 tbspn blancmange (remember, sug sub!) with fresh cream

15. **Fresh or canned salmon, Mixed Salad ("classic")***
    2 oz frozen mousse

16. **Clear soup, Sausage Americana*, cauliflower**
    Coffee Cream Chiffon*

17. **1 small portion beef curry (home-made or canned Brand's)**
    2 rounded tbspn cooked rice, Unflavoured yoghourt

18. **1 portion Salade Niçoise*, 1 apple OR pear, cheese**

19. **Baked fillet of pork, braised celery and 1 carrot**
    1 baked apple (remember—sug sub!) with fresh cream

20. **Casseroled hearts, marrow, green beans**
    6 oz canned strawberries with fresh cream

21. **Spiced Breast of Lamb*, cauliflower, 2 tbspn peas**
    Unflavoured yoghourt OR Coffee Sponge*

22. **Roast best end of neck, 1 roast parsnip, cauliflower**
    Walnut Pear*

23. **Clear soup, Supper Salad***

24. **Kebabs*, cheese and 1 crispbread with butter**

ARE YOU REMEMBERING TO REFER TO
THE BASIC WOMAN DIET RULES, PAGE 133?

high speed weight loss

Question to ask yourself:
Would I find a set routine more simple?

If you answer "yes"—perhaps because you have only a few pounds to lose and repetition would be no problem for you over a short period of time—you will find that this is a diet which is ideal for you in every respect, and the ultimate in swift simplicity.

The simple week's menu can be repeated till you eventually reach your weight loss target.

Refer to the Basic WOMAN Diet Rules on page 133; starred recipes start at page 207.

Monday

Breakfast

Boiled eggs

1 crispbread and butter

Lunch

Ham steaks OR Meat Patty*

2 tbspn peas

Cube of cheese

unflavoured yoghourt

OR junket

Packed lunch

1 crispbread and butter

cheese

Green Salad* (no dressing)

Unflavoured yoghourt

1 small apple

Evening meal

Corned beef OR tongue

2 tbspn canned vegetable salad

1 tomato

2 crispbreads and butter

Tuesday

Breakfast   Ham and poached eggs
1 crispbread and butter

Lunch   Hamburger*
OR frozen Steaklet
OR Beefburger
cabbage
mushrooms
Unflavoured yoghourt
OR baked egg custard
1 apple

Packed lunch   1 crispbread and butter
liver sausage OR luncheon meat
celery
Unflavoured yoghourt
1 small pear

Evening meal   Pair of kippers OR herrings
1 thin slice bread and butter
Coffee Cream Chiffon*

Wednesday

Breakfast

Boiled eggs

1 crispbread and butter

Lunch

Liver and bacon

cauliflower OR cabbage

OR green beans

Stewed pear OR Orange Puffs

with Vanilla Sauce*

Packed lunch

1 crispbread and butter

mashed sardines

OR cream cheese

1 tomato

Unflavoured yoghourt

Evening meal

Ham OR stewed steak

OR minced meat

1 small potato baked in jacket

OR 2 crispbreads and butter

Thursday

Breakfast   Bacon and mushrooms
1 crispbread and butter

Lunch   Braised hearts
OR grilled chops
1 tbspn peas
1 carrot
gherkins
Unflavoured yoghourt

Packed lunch   1 crispbread and butter
cream cheese
cucumber
watercress
1 tangerine
2 oz peanuts
OR 2 oz shelled walnuts

Evening meal   Omelet, Tomato*
Cheese
2 crispbreads and butter

Friday

Breakfast
Scrambled eggs
OR kippers
1 crispbread and butter

Lunch
Steamed or baked fish
Green Salad* OR green beans
Unflavoured yoghourt
OR junket
1 pear

Packed lunch
1 crispbread and butter
corned beef OR hard-boiled egg
1 tomato
watercress
Unflavoured yoghourt

Evening meal
Clear soup
Welsh Rarebit*
raw or cooked celery

Saturday

>>>

Breakfast   Omelet, Bacon*
                       1 crispbread and butter

Lunch   Scotch Egg*
                       OR 2 fried sausages and egg
                       Green Salad* with ½ tomato
                       cheese
                       Unflavoured yoghourt
                       OR Coffee Cream Chiffon*

Evening meal   Clear soup
                       Soft roes OR sardines
                       on 1 thin slice toast

Sunday

>>>

Breakfast   Bacon and egg
                       1 crispbread and butter

Lunch   Roast meat
                       OR Chicken with Lemon Butter*
                       cauliflower OR cabbage
                       2 tbspn fresh fruit salad
                       with fresh cream

Evening meal   Salmon OR crab OR tuna fish
                       Tomato Special*
                       with Green Salad*
                       1 crispbread and butter

AFTER-PREGNANCY DIET

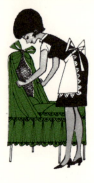

THIS DIET, high in important protein, iron and Vitamin C, is especially designed for new mothers, *after* the breast feeding period, but we do advise the approval of your own doctor. During breast feeding, more carbohydrate is needed to aid the flow of milk, so be sure to take medical advice before you plan any dieting during this period.

Remember to refer to the Basic Rules, page 133, and to use the starred recipes which you will find beginning at page 207.

FIRST WEEK

MONDAY

Breakfast

Grilled Grapefruit*
Boiled eggs
1 slice toast and butter

Lunch

Clear soup
Roes *or* sardines on 1 slice toast, 1 grilled tomato
1 apple *or* orange *or* pear
Unflavoured yoghourt

Evening meal

Meat Parcels*
spinach, cauliflower
4 oz fresh or frozen strawberries with fresh cream
or 1 orange

TUESDAY

Breakfast

Bacon, 1 grilled tomato

Lunch

Omelet, Cheese*
watercress, celery
4 oz grapes *or* 1 apple

Evening meal

Lamb chops
2 tbspn peas, cabbage, 1 sm potato
Apple or gooseberry fool (make as Rhubarb Fool*)
or 1 orange

●

WEDNESDAY

Breakfast

Bacon and mushrooms
1 slice bread and butter

Lunch

Smoked haddock *or* cod, topped with 1 poached egg
1 slice melon (use sug sub if required)
or 1 peach

Evening meal

Mixed grill (liver, kidney, 2 sausages)
cauliflower, 1 grilled tomato
1 sliced pear sprinkled with lemon juice and 1 dspn chopped nuts
or Quickie Pear*

THURSDAY

Breakfast

Scrambled eggs
1 thin slice toast and butter

Lunch

Cauliflower Au Gratin*
Green Salad*
1 apple *or* 1 orange

Evening meal

2 Beefburgers
5 brussels sprouts, 1 grilled tomato
1 slice canned pineapple (*or* 1 pear) with fresh cream

●

FRIDAY

Breakfast

Mushrooms on 1 slice toast
Unflavoured yoghourt

Lunch

$\frac{1}{2}$ grapefruit (use sug sub if required)
Omelet, Tomato*, 2 tbspn peas
Cheese, 1 crispbread and butter

Evening meal

Clear soup
Grilled fish, 2 tbspn broad beans, 1 onion
3 oz fresh blackcurrants (stewed with sug sub) with fresh cream
or 1 orange

SATURDAY

Breakfast

Kippers
1 slice bread and butter

Lunch

Liver and bacon
watercress, Chicory and Caper Salad*
Prune Mousse* *or* 1 pear

Evening meal

Fried chicken
spinach, 2 tbspn sweet corn
2 fresh apricots *or* 1 orange

●

SUNDAY

Breakfast

Bacon and eggs
1 slice toast and butter with 1 tspn marmalade

Lunch

Roast meat
green beans, cauliflower
Coffee Cream Chiffon*

Evening meal

Canned fish
Green Salad*
Cheese, 1 crispbread and butter
Fresh fruit salad (sug sub if required) with fresh cream

MONDAY

Breakfast

Eggs (scrambled with 1 peeled, chopped tomato)
1 slice toast and butter

Lunch

2 sausages, bacon and kidney, cabbage
Unflavoured yoghourt

Evening meal

1 sm pn shepherd's pie, green beans, 1 parsnip
Fruit fool *or* 1 baked apple (sug sub if required)

●

TUESDAY

Breakfast

2 boiled eggs
1 slice bread and butter

Lunch

Clear soup
Fish Fingers, creamed spinach
1 orange *or* 1 pear

Evening meal

Grilled steak, mushrooms, 1 grilled tomato
1 sm potato baked in jacket, with butter
2 oz fresh or frozen raspberries (*or* 1 peach) with fresh cream

WEDNESDAY

Breakfast

Smoked haddock
1 slice bread and butter

Lunch

1 pn Welsh Rarebit*
watercress
4 plums *or* 1 apple

Evening meal

Clear soup
Braised beef
cabbage, 2 tbspn peas
1 *small* portion rice pudding

●

THURSDAY

Breakfast

Poached egg
1 slice toast and butter

Lunch

Salami *or* corned beef
Green Salad*
4 oz grapes *or* 1 apple

Evening meal

Fried chicken
green beans, 2 tbspn sweet corn
2 oz ice-cream

FRIDAY

Breakfast

Tomato Special*
1 slice toast and butter

Lunch

Omelet, Mushroom*
spinach, watercress
2 oz stewed prunes and custard (use sug sub) *or* Prune Mousse*

Evening meal

Clear soup
Grilled white fish, cauliflower, 2 tbspn peas
2 oz frozen mousse *or* 1 peach

●

SATURDAY

Breakfast

Bacon, 2 tbspn baked beans

Lunch

Fried roes *or* pickled herrings
celery, 1 tomato, watercress
1 slice bread and butter
Apple fool (make as Rhubarb Fool*)
or 1 apple chopped in unflavoured yoghourt

Evening meal

Mixed grill (liver, bacon, kidney, 1 sausage, 1 onion)
green beans
1 av pn jelly *or* blancmange

SUNDAY

Breakfast

Bacon and eggs
1 slice toast and butter

Lunch

Roast meat
marrow, cabbage, 1 sm roast potato
2 oz ice-cream

Evening meal

Cold ham *or* meat
Mixed Salad*
1 slice melon (sug sub if required)

THIRD WEEK

MONDAY

Breakfast

Bacon and mushrooms
1 slice toast and butter

Lunch

Chops, spinach, 2 tbspn peas
4 oz cherries *or* 1 apple

Evening meal

Braised beef
1 onion, 1 carrot, green beans
2 tbspn cooked rice pudding and 2 stewed plums (use sug sub)

203

TUESDAY

Breakfast

Scrambled eggs
1 slice toast and butter

Lunch

Liver and onions
braised celery
1 apple *or* 1 orange

Evening meal

Gammon steak
cauliflower, 2 tbspn broad beans
2 oz raspberries (*or* 1 pear) with fresh cream

●

WEDNESDAY
Breakfast

Baked Eggs with Cheese*
1 slice bread and butter

Lunch

Clear soup
Fish Fingers
spinach, 2 tbspn peas
1 orange *or* 1 slice melon

Evening meal

Stewed steak and kidneys
5 brussels sprouts
baked apple and egg custard (use sug sub)

THURSDAY

Breakfast

½ grapefruit (use sug sub if required)
Bacon and mushrooms

Lunch

Stuffed Marrow*
1 sm potato baked in jacket
Walnut Pear*

Evening meal

Golden Hot Pot*
watercress
2 oz ice-cream *or* 2 oz frozen mousse

●

FRIDAY

Breakfast

Unflavoured yoghourt
Kippers *or* boiled eggs
1 slice bread and butter

Lunch

Cauliflower Au Gratin*, Chicory and Caper Salad*
2 halves canned peaches (*or* pears) with fresh cream

Evening meal

Clear soup
Grilled fish *or* Omelet, Mushroom*
green beans, 2 tbspn peas
1 orange

SATURDAY

Breakfast

Scrambled eggs topped with grated cheese
1 slice toast and butter

Lunch

4 frankfurters
French cabbage*, 2 tbspn broad beans
3 oz stewed gooseberries and custard (sug sub for both)
or 1 pear

Evening meal

1 slice melon (sug sub if required)
Fried chicken
5 brussels sprouts
Cheese, 1 crispbread and butter

SUNDAY

Breakfast

Bacon and eggs

Lunch

Roast meat
cauliflower, green beans, 1 sm roast potato
4 oz fresh or frozen strawberries with fresh cream

Evening meal

Cold meat *or* canned fish
Mixed Salad*
1 peach (*or* 1 pear) with 2 oz ice-cream

Woman
SPECIAL-DESIGN RECIPES

NOTE: the recipes are in alphabetical order and, unless otherwise specified, amounts are given for a single portion. These recipes marked ○ are virtually carbohydrate-free and are specially recommended to those who are dieting by Rule of Three or Numbers

APPLE CUPS

SERVES FOUR
4 medium rosy dessert apples
a little lemon juice
Filling:
4 slices cheese
1 tomato
4 spring onions
4 sticks celery
1 green pepper
4 stuffed green olives
4 black olives
8 gherkins
Salad dressing (see Green Salad, page 217)

CUT a thick slice from the top of each apple and slice tops into thin wedges for garnish. Hollow out flesh from apples to make the cup and chop flesh coarsely. Discard the core. Brush the white parts of apple with lemon juice to prevent discoloration. Pile the prepared filling into the apple cups and pour the salad dressing over. Garnish with olives, gherkins and celery leaves.

To prepare filling: cut the cheese into small pieces, the tomato into wedges. Thinly slice the cucumber, wash and chop the celery—reserve the green leaves for garnishing. Trim onions. Slice the peppers. Mix all together with chopped apples.

APRICOT AIRY FAIRY

2 fresh apricots (stoned)
a little water
4 drops sugar substitute
1 egg
knob of butter

COOK apricots in a little water with 2 drops sugar substitute till tender. Mash with a fork until a smooth pulp. Separate egg. Beat yolk lightly. Whisk egg white till stiff, and divide into two. Add sugar substitute to one half and leave on one side for topping. Add other half to yolk and blend quickly and lightly together. Melt butter in frying pan. Add egg mixture in a round. When golden brown, turn over and cook other side.
Spread egg round with apricot purée, top with remaining whisked egg white and brown quickly under the grill.

O BAKED EGGS WITH CHEESE

2 oz grated Cheddar cheese
2 eggs
salt
pepper

PLACE 1 oz cheese in the base of a greased individual oven-proof dish. Break the eggs into the dish, season to taste and sprinkle with the remaining cheese. Bake in a moderate oven (350 deg. F—Mark 4) for 10 minutes.

BUCK RAREBIT

SERVES THREE
Welsh Rarebit (see page 232)
3 eggs

MAKE Welsh Rarebit, top each slice with a poached egg.

CAULIFLOWER AU GRATIN

SERVES TWO
1 small cauliflower
3 oz grated cheese
½ pint white sauce

COOK and drain cauliflower, put in greased fireproof dish. Add 2 oz grated cheese to hot white sauce. Pour sauce over cauliflower. Top with rest of cheese. Brown under grill.

O CAULIFLOWER SAVOURY

½ small cauliflower
½ oz butter
1 onion
1 tomato
salt
pepper

BREAK the cauliflower into sprigs and cook till tender in a saucepan with a little boiling salted water. Drain. Meanwhile melt butter in saucepan, add the peeled, chopped onion. Cook till tender, add peeled, diced tomato, salt and pepper. Stir well, and cook for another 5 minutes or till really soft. Pour over cauliflower in serving dish.

CHEESEY EGGS

2 hard-boiled eggs
¼ pint white sauce
1 oz grated cheese

PLACE the halved hard-boiled eggs in a greased fireproof dish. Cover with the white sauce. Sprinkle grated cheese on top and grill until top is golden brown and bubbling.

CHEESE SANDWICH SOUFFLE

1 thin slice bread
1 slice cheese
2 eggs
1 dessertspoon mayonnaise
pinch salt

TOAST the slice of bread on one side. Cover the untoasted side with a slice of cheese. Separate whites and yolks of eggs, add mayonnaise to yolks and beat. Add salt to whites and whisk till stiff then fold in yolks mixture. Pile onto cheese. Bake in a moderate oven (350 deg. F—Mark 4) about 15 minutes.

○ CHICKEN WITH LEMON BUTTER

SERVES FOUR
4 chicken joints
salt
pepper
3 oz butter
1 tablespoon oil
juice of 1 lemon
2 bayleaves
chopped parsley
lemon slices

WIPE the chicken and season well. Heat 2 oz butter with the oil in frying pan and fry the joints till golden brown all over and cooked through, about 15–20 minutes. Place the chicken on a hot serving dish and keep hot. Add remaining butter to the pan and when hot add the lemon juice and the bay leaves and boil for a short while. Pour over the chicken, sprinkle with parsley and garnish with lemon slices.

○ CHICORY AND CAPER SALAD

1 head of chicory
1 teaspoon chopped capers
1 dessertspoon sour cream or unflavoured yoghourt

SLICE the chicory into thin rings. Mix with the capers and the sour cream or yoghourt.
To garnish, top with chopped parsley.

○ COD EN COCOTTE

1 small onion
1 oz butter
1 cod cutlet
salt
pepper
slices of tomato
1 oz grated cheese

PEEL and chop the onion and fry in melted butter. Place it in the bottom of a fireproof dish. Put cod cutlet on top of onion, season, surround with slices of tomato. Sprinkle with grated cheese. Bake in a moderate oven (350 deg. F—Mark 4) for 20–30 minutes.

○ COFFEE CREAM CHIFFON

¼ **pint double cream**
a little sugar substitute
instant coffee

WHIP cream until stiff, add a little sugar substitute and the instant coffee to taste. Whip again, chill and serve.

○ COFFEE SPONGE

SERVES TWO
¼ **pint black coffee**
½ **oz gelatine**
¼ **pint milk**
½ **teaspoon vanilla essence**
1–2 drops sugar substitute
2 egg whites

PLACE black coffee and gelatine in a small pan and heat until gelatine has dissolved. Add milk, vanilla essence and sugar substitute and pour into bowl. When almost set whisk in stiffly beaten egg whites. Chill. Serve with fresh cream.

○ CUCUMBER GALA PLATTER

SERVES TWO
4 hard-boiled eggs
4 oz cottage cheese
salt
pepper
½ cucumber
¼ pint double cream
1 tablespoon milk
6 black olives

SHELL and chop the hard-boiled eggs, mix with cottage cheese and season to taste. Thinly slice the cucumber. Whip the cream with the milk till stiff. Pile the egg in the centre of a plate and arrange the cucumber around the edge. Pipe the cream in a circle between the egg and cucumber and a little in the centre. Garnish with the olives.

DANISH MEAT BALLS

1 onion
2 oz minced veal or beef
½ egg
salt
pepper
a little flour
1 oz butter

MINCE or grate peeled onion. Mix with raw minced veal or beef and bind with beaten egg. Season. Form into oval shapes and lightly coat with flour. Fry in hot butter on both sides until brown and sufficiently cooked.

○ ESCALOP OF VEAL WITH CHEESE

1 escalop of veal
1 oz butter
1 slice cheese

FRY the escalop in butter. Approximately 5 minutes before it is ready, top with a slice of cheese and fry for a few more minutes, so that the cheese melts slightly.

○ FRENCH CABBAGE

2 onions
1 oz butter
¼ cabbage
2 tablespoons water
salt
pepper

PEEL and slice the onion and cook in the melted butter till tender. Add the sliced cabbage, water, and seasoning to taste. Cover and simmer *gently* till tender, 7–10 minutes, shaking pan occasionally. Half a lettuce may be used instead of the cabbage, if liked. Can be served with tomatoes.

○ GOLDEN HOT POT

1 small onion
2 oz mushrooms
6 oz middle neck of lamb
salt
pepper
$\frac{1}{4}$ pint stock

PLACE alternate layers of sliced onion, mushrooms and middle neck of lamb in fireproof dish, seasoning well between layers. Pour in stock, cover with kitchen foil and cook in moderately slow oven (335 deg. F—Mark 3) for about 1$\frac{1}{2}$ hours or till tender.

○ GREEN SALAD

lettuce
cucumber
watercress
cabbage
Dressing:
pinch of salt
pepper
1 tablespoon oil
1 dessertspoon vinegar

SHRED or chop raw vegetables and toss well together in dressing. *To make salad dressing:* place salt, pepper, oil and vinegar in a screw-topped jar and shake well till thoroughly blended.

GRILLED GRAPEFRUIT

½ grapefruit
few drops sugar substitute

SPRINKLE the half grapefruit with sugar substitute. Place under medium grill for about 5 minutes. Serve hot.

O HAM AND EGG HUMPIES

¼ lb chopped lean ham
chopped parsley
2 eggs
salt
pepper

LIGHTLY BRUSH small mould with oil and one-third fill with the ham and parsley. Break eggs into the mould and stand it in a pan of boiling water to come half-way up sides of mould. Season to taste. Cover pan and cook until the eggs are set; serve hot.

OHAMBURGER

3 oz raw minced beef
1 teaspoon chopped onion
salt
pepper
a little beaten egg for binding
fat for frying

MIX beef with onion. Season and add sufficient egg to bind the mixture together. Shape into small flat round. Fry in hot fat for a few minutes on each side until brown and tender.

HAWAIIAN CIRCLE

1 thick slice gammon
1 ring canned pineapple
2–3 oz grated cheese

PLACE ham steak topped with pineapple and grated cheese in small greased oven-proof dish. Bake in a moderately hot oven (375 deg. F—Mark 5) for about 30 minutes or until ham is cooked through.

O KEBABS

uncooked meat (any)
button or quartered mushrooms
green pepper
2 quartered tomatoes
salt
pepper

THREAD small cubes of uncooked meat, a few mushrooms, pieces of green pepper and quartered tomatoes on to skewer, season and brush with oil. Place under medium grill until cooked, turning frequently.

KEDGEREE

1 tablespoon cooked rice
2 oz butter
4 oz cooked, flaked white fish
2 hard-boiled eggs
pepper

PUT rice in small pan with the melted butter. Stir over a gentle heat until thoroughly re-heated. Add the fish and chopped hard-boiled eggs. Season lightly with pepper. Mix well and serve hot.

MAXIMILIENNE EGGS

2 large tomatoes
salt
pepper
2 eggs
grated cheese

CUT tops off tomatoes and scoop out centre. Season. Drop an egg into each tomato, pile on grated cheese. Bake in a moderate oven (350 deg. F—Mark 4) for about 20 minutes or until eggs are set.

MEAT PARCELS

4 oz cooked minced meat
2 teaspoons chopped onion
salt
pepper
a little beaten egg
flour for binding
2 bacon rashers
fat for frying

MIX cooked mince with finely chopped onion. Season to taste and bind with beaten egg and flour; shape into two patties. Wrap each inside a bacon rasher. Secure with wooden cocktail sticks. Fry in shallow fat, turning till golden brown. Remove sticks and serve.

MEAT PATTY

2 oz cooked minced meat (fresh or leftovers)
1 teaspoon chopped onion
chopped parsley
salt
pepper
a little beaten egg for binding
½ teaspoon flour
1 bacon rasher

MIX minced meat with peeled and finely chopped onion and chopped parsley. Season to taste and bind together with beaten egg and flour. Shape into 1 in. round patty. Remove rind from bacon rasher and wrap rasher round patty. Secure with wooden cocktail stick. Grill patty until golden brown.

○ MIXED SALAD

"Classic" ingredients:
lettuce
tomato
cucumber
radishes
spring onions
salad dressing (see Green Salad, page 217)

Suggested additions or variations:
sliced or grated beetroot
grated carrot
cabbage
sliced orange
sliced apple
endive
chicory

SHRED or chop ingredients as necessary and mix well with the salad dressing. Most people have their own preferences and quickly develop a liking for particular salad ingredients.

MUSHROOM SAUCE

2 oz mushrooms
½ oz butter
2 teaspoons flour
1 teaspoon paprika
¼ pint cold milk

FRY mushrooms gently in melted butter. Mix the flour and paprika with the milk. Add to mushrooms and bring to the boil; stir until mixture thickens. Simmer a few minutes.

○ OMELET, SAVOURY

2 eggs
1 tablespoon water
salt
pepper
$\frac{1}{2}$ oz butter
Fillings:
1 oz grated cheese ○
OR 1 oz chopped ham ○
OR 1 peeled, diced tomato
OR 2 rashers bacon, chopped and fried till crisp ○
OR 2 oz mushrooms, peeled, sliced and gently fried ○
OR $\frac{1}{2}$ lb fresh spinach, washed, shaken dry and cooked without extra water till soft ○

WHISK the eggs with the water and seasoning to taste. Heat the fat in a small frying or omelet pan, pour in the egg and cook, stirring the mixture lightly with the back of a fork till the omelet is lightly set. Add the prepared filling and fold the omelet in half.

OMELET, SWEET

2 eggs
1 dessertspoon jam
a little water

MAKE a plain omelet as for Savoury Omelet, omitting the seasoning, and sweeten with a sauce made from 1 dessertspoon of jam warmed with a little water to thin.

ORANGE PUFFS WITH VANILLA SAUCE

SERVES TWO
2 eggs, separated
8 drops sugar substitute
2 drops vanilla essence
10 tablespoons milk
1 orange, peeled and cut into segments

BEAT the egg yolks with 4 drops of the sugar substitute and the vanilla essence. Bring the milk to the boil and whisk into the yolks. Return the mixture to the pan and cook very slowly, stirring all the time, till the mixture coats the back of the spoon—do not allow to boil. Pour the sauce into two individual oven-proof dishes. Whisk the egg whites with the remaining sugar substitute till stiff, then fold in the chopped orange segments. Divide the mixture between the two dishes and place under a medium hot grill to brown. Serve hot.

PRINCESS SOUFFLE

1 oz dried apricots
2 oz cooking apple
5 drops sugar substitute
1 egg white

SOAK apricots overnight; simmer in a little water till nearly cooked, add peeled and sliced apple and 3 drops sugar substitute. Simmer till tender. Drain off any excess juice, sieve. Whip egg white with 2 drops sugar substitute until very stiff. Fold into sieved fruit. Put into individual greased baking dish and cook in moderate oven (350 deg. F—Mark 4) for 10 minutes or until well-risen and cooked. Serve at once.

PRUNE MOUSSE

3 oz dried prunes
weak tea (without milk)
½ slice lemon
4 drops sugar substitute
1 level teaspoon gelatine
1 egg white
1 drop almond essence

SOAK prunes overnight. Cook gently in tea with lemon and 2 drops sugar substitute until soft. Drain off juice (add water if necessary to make up to 2 tablespoons); heat, and dissolve gelatine in it. Stone prunes and sieve together with juice, leave to cool. Whisk egg white with 2 drops sugar substitute. Fold in purée gradually—the mixture must be light. Add drop of almond essence and beat well. Put into glass dish and leave to set.

QUICKIE PEAR

1 egg
2 drops sugar substitute
1 drop almond essence
1 medium pear
1 oz chopped walnuts
1 teaspoon chopped raisins

WHISK white of egg with sugar substitute and almond essence until stiff. Peel, halve and core pear and fill hollows with chopped walnuts mixed with the chopped raisins. Pile the meringue mixture on top of the pears and brown in a moderately hot oven (375 deg. F—Mark 5) for about 5 minutes.

○ RHUBARB FOOL

1 portion of stewed rhubarb (unsweetened)
2–3 drops sugar substitute
2 tablespoons fresh cream or unflavoured yoghourt

MASH the portion of stewed rhubarb with the drops of sugar substitute and mix with the cream or unflavoured yoghourt. Chill well, if possible, before serving.

○ SALADE NIÇOISE

SERVES TWO
1 hearty lettuce
1 medium onion
2 tomatoes
2 hard-boiled eggs
1 small can anchovy fillets
8 black olives
Dressing:
4 tablespoons oil
2 tablespoons vinegar
salt
pepper
parsley

WASH lettuce and tear into pieces. Peel and thinly slice the onion, cut the tomato into wedges. Shell the eggs and cut into chunks. Toss all the prepared ingredients together with the anchovy fillets, black olives and the salad dressing. Serve at once.

To prepare dressing: place all the ingredients in a screw-topped jar and shake till thoroughly blended.

SAUCY PUDDING

2 oz cooking apple
1 dessertspoon water
2 drops sugar substitute
¼ oz butter
good pinch cinnamon (or to taste)
1 slice bread
1 tablespoon beaten egg
knob of butter

PEEL and core the apple and slice thinly, add water and the sugar substitute. Cook over a low heat. Put apple in a small basin, add butter and cinnamon and beat until smooth. Soak bread on both sides in beaten egg (if bread is stale, a whole egg can be used). Warm a frying pan, melt butter and fry bread on both sides till golden brown. Put bread on a heated plate and spread with the apple mixture.

SAUSAGE AMERICANA

4 chipolata sausages
fat for frying
2 oz mushrooms
1 small can tomato purée
pinch curry powder

FRY sausages in melted fat until golden brown. Remove from pan. Slice mushrooms, fry till tender. Drain off excess fat, add tomato purée, a pinch of curry powder and seasoning. Place the sausages in sauce. Cook gently for 10 minutes.

SCOTCH EGG

1 small egg
2 oz sausage meat
a little flour
egg for binding
breadcrumbs
fat for deep frying

BOIL egg hard and shell it. Roll or pat out sausage meat into a round. Dip egg in flour and fold sausage meat round it, and seal well. Brush with beaten egg, roll in breadcrumbs and fry in deep fat until golden brown. Serve hot or cold.

○ SPICED BREAST OF LAMB

SERVES FOUR
1 boned rolled breast of lamb
1 small onion
salt
pepper
mixed herbs

PUT lamb in water to cover with onion, seasoning, and mixed herbs tied in muslin. Simmer for $1\frac{1}{2}$–2 hours or until tender. Remove herbs. Serve the meat cut into slices. (Liquid may be drunk as a clear soup.)

○ STUFFED MARROW

½ small onion
¼ lb minced beef
3 tablespoons unthickened gravy
salt
pepper
1 in. thick slice vegetable marrow
½ oz grated cheese

FRY peeled, chopped onion. Add minced beef; cook quickly, stirring until brown. Add gravy; cook, covered, 15–20 minutes, stirring occasionally. Season to taste. Discard seeds from slice of marrow, place in buttered fireproof dish. Fill centre with mince, top with grated cheese; bake in moderately hot oven (375 deg. F—Mark 5) for 30 minutes, until cheese has lightly browned.

○ STUFFED PEPPERS

1 onion
¼ lb. minced beef
3 tablespoons unthickened gravy
salt
pepper
1 green pepper
½ oz grated cheese

FRY peeled, chopped onion, add minced beef and cook quickly, stirring occasionally. Add gravy, cover and cook gently for 20 minutes. Season. Halve green pepper, remove top and seeds. Parboil 5 minutes. Drain. Fill halves with mince. Bake, covered with foil, in moderate oven (350 deg. F—Mark 4) for about 30 minutes. Remove foil. Top with grated cheese, bake another 10 minutes.

SUPPER SALAD

1 dessert apple
lemon juice
2 oz cold ham
1 small sliced green pepper
1 tablespoon sour cream or unflavoured yoghourt
1 tablespoon top of milk
lettuce leaves
1 oz crumbled blue cheese
sliced tomato
sliced cucumber

CORE and dice the eating apple. Sprinkle with lemon juice. Mix with cold ham and green pepper. Blend sour cream or yoghourt with top of milk, add to prepared mixture and toss well together. Pile in bowl lined with lettuce leaves, sprinkle with the crumbled cheese and garnish with sliced tomato and cucumber.

○ TOMATO SPECIAL

1 medium tomato
$\frac{1}{2}$ oz cheese

HALVE the tomato, grate the cheese and pile it on to tomato halves. Cook quickly under the grill till cheese browns slightly.

VEGETABLE PLATE

A.
1 small carrot, thinly sliced
1 portion cabbage, sliced
1 boiled onion
1 stick celery
1 cooked beetroot
1 grilled tomato

B.
1 portion marrow slices
1 leek cut into rings
3 oz brussels sprouts
1 sm pn turnips or parsnips
1 portion spinach
1 grilled tomato

ARRANGE mixed cooked vegetables attractively on a dish. They can be either steamed or poached in a little water. Probably the easiest method is to steam a selection of vegetables together. The dish should be served without liquid, so include a baked or grilled tomato as a form of sauce. Serve sprinkled with chopped chives or parsley. Two variations are given above, or you can make your own selection.

VEGETABLE STEW

selection of chopped or diced raw vegetables, e.g.:
carrots
turnip
onions
leeks
2–3 slices red or green peppers
2 skinned tomatoes
1 pint canned or fresh tomato juice or a Marmite gravy
salt
pepper

PLACE all the prepared vegetables in a saucepan with the tomato juice or gravy and seasoning to taste. Cover the pan and simmer gently for about 1 hour until the vegetables are tender.

WALNUT PEAR

1 medium pear
unflavoured yoghourt or whipped cream
1 oz chopped walnuts

PEEL, halve and core the pear, fill hollows with yoghourt or whipped cream and top with the chopped walnuts. Serve at once.

WELSH RAREBIT

SERVES THREE
4 oz grated Cheddar cheese
a little milk
$\frac{1}{4}$ level teaspoon made mustard
pepper
3 thin slices buttered toast

MIX the cheese with enough milk to bind, made mustard and pepper to taste. Divide the mixture between the slices of toast and spread out evenly. Place under a hot grill and cook till topping is golden brown.

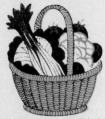

SHOPPING CALENDAR

NOWADAYS, with improved methods of production, storage and transport, you can buy almost any food at any time of the year (see below) but the cost varies greatly. On the following pages we give you some indication of the economical times to buy some of the common foods you will want to keep an eye on, plus a few exotic items for occasional extravagance. We show you when either they are at their best or, because they are home-grown and not imported, they are cheapest. Remember that this is a rough guide only and that local produce in the north of England and Scotland may at times be anything up to a month later than the south to reach its peak.

SOME FOODS READILY AVAILABLE THROUGHOUT THE YEAR

(Remember, you can get almost anything at any time—at a price)

FRUITS — Apples, avocado pears, bananas, grapefruit, grapes, lemons, oranges, pineapples

VEGETABLES AND SALAD — Beetroot, broccoli, cabbage, carrots, cauliflower, globe artichokes, horseradish, leeks, lettuce, mushrooms, mustard and cress, onions, parsley, radishes, spinach, tomatoes, turnips, watercress

MEATS — Beef, veal, lamb (English lamb shown in calendar), chicken

FISH — Bream, brill, cod, crayfish, dory, eels, haddock, hake, halibut, mullet, mussels, plaice, prawns, salmon (imported), shrimps, sole, turbot, whiting

NOW TURN THE PAGE FOR THE MONTH-BY-MONTH BEST BUYING TIMES

JANUARY
FRUITS   Cooking apples, imported apples and pears

VEGETABLES   Artichokes (Jerusalem), brussels sprouts, celeriac, celery,
AND SALAD   chicory, kale, parsnips

MEATS   Duck, goose, lamb, pork, rabbit, turkey

FISH   Herrings, mackerel, oysters, scallops, sprats

FEBRUARY
FRUITS   Cooking apples, imported apples and pears

VEGETABLES   Artichokes (Jerusalem), brussels sprouts, celeriac, celery,
AND SALAD   chicory, kale, parsnips

MEATS   Duck, goose, lamb, pork, turkey

FISH   Herrings, mackerel, oysters, scallops, sprats

MARCH
FRUITS   Rhubarb, imported apples and pears

VEGETABLES   Artichokes (Jerusalem), aubergines, brussels sprouts,
AND SALAD   celeriac, chicory, kale, parsnips, turnip tops

MEATS   Duck, duckling, lamb, pork

FISH   Mackerel, oysters, scallops, sprats, whitebait

APRIL
FRUITS   Rhubarb, imported apples and pears

VEGETABLES   Aubergines, parsnips, turnip tops, young greens
AND SALAD

MEATS   Duckling, lamb

FISH   Mackerel, oysters, scallops, sprats, whitebait

MAY

FRUITS	Cherries, cherry plums, gooseberries, rhubarb
VEGETABLES AND SALAD	Asparagus, aubergines, beans (broad), young greens
MEATS	Duckling, gosling, lamb
FISH	Crab, mackerel, whitebait

JUNE

FRUITS	Apricots, cherries, cherry plums, blackcurrants, gooseberries, peaches, redcurrants, rhubarb, strawberries (beginning)
VEGETABLES AND SALAD	Asparagus, aubergines, beans (broad), cucumbers (English), peas, peppers (green) tomatoes (English beginning)
MEATS	Duck, gosling, lamb
FISH	Crab, mackerel, whitebait

JULY

FRUITS	Apricots, cherries, gooseberries, greengages, peaches, plums (English), raspberries, strawberries
VEGETABLES AND SALAD	Asparagus, aubergines, beans (broad and runner), cucumbers (English), marrow, peas, peppers (green), tomatoes (English), young greens
MEATS	Duck, gosling, lamb
FISH	Crab, herrings, salmon (British), whitebait

AUGUST

FRUITS	Blackberries, blackcurrants, greengages, melons, peaches, raspberries, plums (English), strawberries
VEGETABLES AND SALAD	Aubergines, beans (runner), cucumber (English), brussels sprouts, marrow, parsnips, peas, peppers (green and red), tomatoes (English), young greens
MEATS	Duck, grouse, hare
FISH	Crab, herrings, salmon (British), whitebait

SEPTEMBER

FRUITS | Apples (English), blackberries, melons, pears (English)

VEGETABLES AND SALAD | Artichokes (Jerusalem), aubergines, celeriac, celery, chicory, cucumbers (English), marrow, parsnips, peppers (green and red), pumpkin, tomatoes (English)

MEATS | Duck, goose, grouse, rabbit, pork

FISH | Crab, herrings, oysters

OCTOBER

FRUITS | Apples (English), blackberries, pears (English)

VEGETABLES AND SALAD | Artichokes (Jerusalem), aubergines, brussels sprouts, celeriac, celery, chicory, cucumbers (English), endive, kale, marrow, parsnips, peppers (green and red), pumpkin, young greens

MEATS | Duck, goose, pork, rabbit, turkey

FISH | Herrings, oysters, scallops

NOVEMBER

FRUITS | Cooking apples (English), pears (English, ending)

VEGETABLES AND SALAD | Artichokes (Jerusalem), celeriac, celery, chicory, endive, kale, parsnips, peppers (red), young greens

MEATS | Duck, goose, pork, rabbit, turkey

FISH | Herrings, mackerel, oysters, scallops, sprats

DECEMBER

FRUITS | Cooking apples, imported apples and pears

VEGETABLES AND SALAD | Artichokes (Jerusalem), brussels sprouts, celeriac, celery, chicory, endive, kale, parsnips, peppers (red), young greens

MEATS | Duck, goose, pork, turkey

FISH | Herrings, mackerel, oysters, scallops, sprats

INDEX

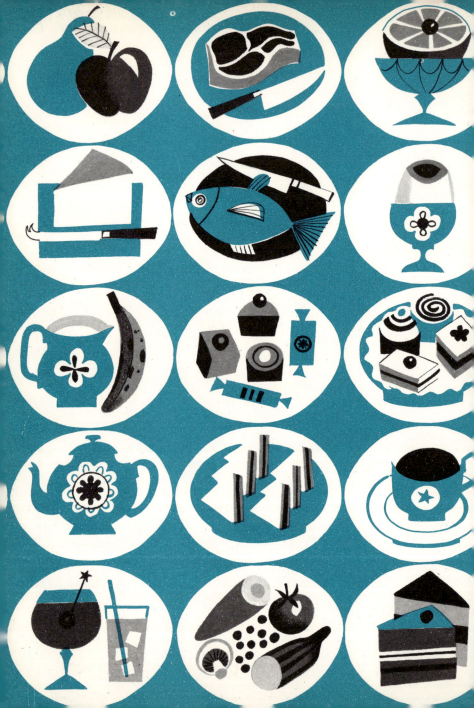